The Mediterranean Diet

Eric Zacharias, M.D.

The Mediterranean Diet

A Clinician's Guide for Patient Care

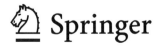 Springer

Eric Zacharias, M.D.
Chairman, Department of Medicine, Boulder Medical Center
Assistant Clinical Professor, University of Colorado Health Sciences Center
2750 Broadway
Boulder, Colorado
USA

Additional material to this book can be downloaded from http://extras.springer.com.

ISBN 978-1-4614-3325-5   ISBN 978-1-4614-3326-2 (eBook)
DOI 10.1007/978-1-4614-3326-2
Springer New York Heidelberg Dordrecht London

Library of Congress Control Number: 2012934830

Springer is part of Springer Science+Business Media (www.springer.com)

To my colleagues in all fields of clinical care who strive every day to promote health in their patients.

Preface

For what is likely the first time in the history of mankind, our health is more threatened by easy access to food—specifically, high calorie density and low nutrient density food—than by food scarcity. The fact that many individuals in our modern society, perhaps even the majority, over-eat unhealthy foods is a common observation, and there are frequent reports in both the professional and lay media of the dramatic worldwide rise in obesity and other morbidity directly related to our diet. A promising counterpoint to the nearly universal trend of the developed world's worsening dietary pattern is the increasing popularity of one common pattern of eating that has actually been shown to reduce rates of disease and obesity and to promote longevity—a Mediterranean diet. As an Internal Medicine specialist I have devoted my professional and personal life to investigating diet for health promotion and longevity; I have been encouraged by the scientific research that consistently shows the health benefits of a Mediterranean diet. My interest in this topic led me to spend a 6-month sabbatical researching the Mediterranean diet and lifestyle at its origins in the countries bordering the Mediterranean Sea. This book is a summary of my research on the critical topic of how, in a world where unhealthy food options abound, a Mediterranean diet may be a powerful tool to help reverse the obesity and disease trends directly related to unhealthy eating.

Colorado, USA   Eric Zacharias, MD

Acknowledgments

There are many individuals who helped me at the various stages of this book.

For the initial inspiration, brain storming, and book proposal review—Mickey Haynes, John Sergent, Andy Pruitt, Alex Bogusky, and Benjy Mikel and the Department of Food Science, Nutrition, and Health Promotion at Mississippi State University.

For the approval of and logistics for a sabbatical in the Mediterranean countries—The physicians of the Boulder Medical Center, Sarah Zacharias, Katherine Zacharias, and Luke Zacharias.

For research assistance—Angela Fredrickson and Margaret Fletcher.

For recipe testing and evaluation—J. Hill, Amanda Louey, Tara Raposo, Kim Moss, Patrick Green, Greg Faith, Joanna Faith, Gordon Tanner, Anna Tanner, Karl Maier, Julie Maier, Ben Moss, Angela McGrath, Tim Lindholm, Tommie Zacharias, Donald Lancaster, Hilary Lancaster, Karen Savage, Alex Preiser, Leslie Zacharias, Thomas Landry, Charles Corfield, Steve Hartley, Mindy Hartley, David Packard, LaDawn Oliver, Bobbi Watt, Eric Sorenson, Jeannine Fox, Scott Reardon, Sue Reardon, Alan Zacharias, Robert O'Herron, Jane O'Herron, Walt Wehner, Sarah Altschuler, Kim Mugler, Jennie Smith, Andrew Biglow, Heather Biglow, Caroline Landry, Tiphaine Bonetti, Paolo Bonetti, Scot Thigpen, Kimberly Inkster Thigpen, David Kirk, Molly Kirk, Katherine Zacharias, Luke Zacharias, Sarah Zacharias.

For serving as this book's invaluable development editor—Maureen Pierce.

Contents

Part I
The Basics of a Mediterranean Diet

Chapter 1
Introduction

Let food be thy medicine and medicine be thy food.

Hippocrates (ca. 460 BC–ca. 370 BC)

Keywords Mediterranean diet • Health benefits • Weight loss • Realistic diet • Time constraints

"What is the best diet for my health?" This is one of the most common and important questions healthcare providers are asked, and yet a simple and concise answer can be elusive. There is no one "best diet," but, of the myriad dietary strategies that have been studied over the years, the data presented in this book show that a Mediterranean diet (MedDiet) clearly is an excellent option. Three themes are expanded on regarding this diet: First, a MedDiet is proven to be good for health. Hundreds of clinical trials are cited, involving hundreds of thousands of individual patients who have demonstrated its effects in reducing cardiovascular disease, cancer, diabetes, Alzheimer's disease, controlling weight, and increasing quality and quantity of life. Second, a Mediterranean diet is effective for weight loss and control. A MedDiet is not exclusively a "diet" as traditionally held in the American vernacular meaning "eating to lose weight." It has been chiefly studied and promoted due to strong evidence that it improves health and reduces disease risk. However, the data summarized demonstrate that a MedDiet is at least as effective for weight loss as any other diet. Weight loss and control is of great interest to many patients for both their health and general appearance, so substantial information is provided on this topic. Additionally, the new Medicare benefit covering "screening and counseling for obesity" is summarized. The third major theme is that a MedDiet is simultaneously delicious and realistic to implement into a busy American lifestyle. There are many reasons that most attempts at dieting for health and weight control fail in the long-term, but overly rigorous demands of adherents and lack of palatability are two common ones. Food plays a central role in life, and in this book a MedDiet is shown to be easy to implement

E. Zacharias, *The Mediterranean Diet: A Clinician's Guide for Patient Care*,
DOI 10.1007/978-1-4614-3326-2_1, © Springer Science+Business Media, LLC 2012

and congruous with the pleasure and lifestyle most patients associate with good food. By offering examples of ways to gather, prepare, and eat food in a more healthy fashion, this book will help clinicians work with patients to craft a sustainable and healthy dietary strategy. Food's taste, convenience of preparation, and acceptability to any given situation is paramount to long-term dietary compliance. The MedDiet originated from cultures that love food, and food for optimal health or weight loss and food for pleasure and convenience are not mutually exclusive.

This book is written for healthcare providers as both a summary of the health benefits of a Mediterranean Diet and as a guide to sharing science-based nutrition information, practical meal plans, and healthy recipes with patients. It is reasonable to ask how well we are doing as a nation with the books and dietary strategies we currently use for disease prevention. In the diseases section, data are presented that show we are in the midst of obesity and diabetes epidemics in both children and adults, and our current generation of children threatens to be the first in modern times to not have life expectancies greater than their parents. This is directly related to changes in our diets and lifestyles over the past 40 years. As a healthcare provider, it is hard to not be discouraged by this abysmal assessment, but it also shows that there is significant room and need for a more successful approach. In today's practice environment, dominated by brief clinic appointments, it can be challenging for clinicians to add discussions about dietary strategies to the time already spent addressing other health concerns. As a busy primary care provider who deals with these real-world time constraints daily, I have aimed to make this book an office instrument that I would find useful in my practice.

Although the need for an improved diet in the United States is clear, accomplishing this has been elusive. An area of particular interest of mine is improving effectiveness at the provider level. My experience from tens of thousands of patient clinic visits has revealed several barriers that need to be overcome. First, in-depth discussion about diet is time consuming. Also, the effects of improvements in diet on disease risk reduction may take years or even decades to become apparent. For example, the benefits of preventing hundreds of myocardial infarctions, strokes, cases of diabetes, and other diseases through preventive health care are not as immediately obvious as saving the life of a single individual having an acute myocardial infarction. This lack of any near-term positive results, especially for chronic diseases, can make counseling seem less immediately important than addressing acute patient illnesses. Both are surely important. In addition, our current healthcare system reimburses more generously for procedures and treatment of diseases already present than for the cognitive services and time involved in helping with their prevention. This book may assist clinicians to overcome these barriers in the following ways:

- A reliable book to recommend to patients for further reading should help with the office time constraints.
- The data showing the power of long-term disease reduction by a MedDiet may help in making the benefits of compliance seem more tangible.

- As more providers and patients become tuned to the health benefits and cost savings of disease prevention by diet and lifestyle, government and private insurance payers may take notice and start to reimburse these efforts at a level that reflects their true impact on outcomes.

Information Presented

When summarizing studies regarding a MedDiet presented in this book, primary references are used for the majority of information presented, and these may be searched if further review is desired. Large, high-quality, meta-analyses have been published on some topics, and these are cited when appropriate. Lastly, the 2010 Dietary Guidelines for Americans Advisory Committee (DGAC, 2010) is cited as a reference on several important topics [1]. It is an authoritative group of many of the nation's leading nutrition scientists convened every 5 years by the US Department of Agriculture and the US Department of Health and Human Services to publish current consensus on important health questions based on comprehensive reviews of the published scientific literature.

This book is organized into two main sections.

Section 1

First, the history, foods, and consumption patterns of a MedDiet are explained. The specific nutrients in the diet and an explanation of how a MedDiet adherence score is calculated and used in clinical studies are included. Next, the effects of a MedDiet on overall mortality and compression of morbidity as well as on common diseases including cardiovascular diseases, cancer, Alzheimer's, diabetes, obesity, asthma, and allergic and autoimmune conditions are detailed. Information about the epidemiology of obesity in the United States and the use of a MedDiet as a safe, healthy, and effective dietary approach for controlling weight follows. A patient encounter form designed to be used in the exam room when providing patients the new Medicare covered benefit of "screening and counseling for obesity" is included. Lastly, nutrition information is provided on the macronutrients in a MedDiet including basic biochemical and physiologic information about dietary proteins, carbohydrates, lipids, and alcohol.

Section 2

This section serves to assist with the practical implementation of a MedDiet. It contains templates for daily meal recommendations that follow the principles of a MedDiet along with a large recipe section to help with preparing delicious and healthy Mediterranean meals at home.

Reference

1. Dietary Guidelines for Americans Advisory Committee (DGAC) 2010. U.S. Department of Agriculture. Center for Nutrition Policy and Promotion. Dietary guidelines for Americans 2010. http://www.cnpp.usda.gov/dietaryguidelines.htm. Accessed 1 Jan 2011.

Chapter 2
History, Composition, Adherence Scores

Keywords Mediterranean diet • Seven countries study • Saturated fat • Unsaturated fat • Mediterranean diet pyramid • Adherence

Defining a Mediterranean Diet

The term "Mediterranean diet" is commonly used to refer to the historic dietary pattern consumed by the population of the Mediterranean regions in the 1950s and 1960s, which was associated with extremely low rates of coronary heart disease (CHD) and mortality. MedDiet also refers to an idealized and quantifiable dietary pattern developed by nutrition scientists that is derived from this original diet. In the 1950s, nutrition scientists observed a significant geographic disparity in the rates of cardiovascular diseases and mortality in the developed world. Specifically, populations in the olive-growing regions of Southern Europe had lower CHD rates and longer life expectancies than populations in Northern Europe and the United States [1–5]. They evaluated variables in the dietary patterns of these regions in an attempt to find an element or elements responsible for these differences (Fig. 2.1).

The most well-known study to investigate the health impacts of diet was the Seven Countries study. Initiated in the 1960s, the Seven Countries study observed that although populations of the Mediterranean region, Northern Europe, and the United States all had relatively high dietary fat intakes, the sources of fats being consumed were different. The Northern European and US populations obtained fat chiefly from saturated fat of animal origin, and the Mediterranean-region Europeans obtained fat chiefly from unsaturated fat of plant origin, with olive oil being particularly common. After 20 years of epidemiologic observations, the Seven Countries study investigators reported that both all-cause and CHD death rates were positively associated with percentage of dietary energy obtained from saturated fatty acids and were negatively

Regional Differences in Coronary Heart Disease in the 1960s

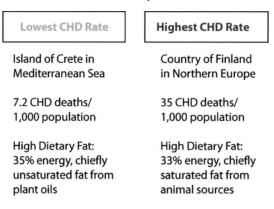

Lowest CHD Rate	Highest CHD Rate
Island of Crete in Mediterranean Sea	Country of Finland in Northern Europe
7.2 CHD deaths/ 1,000 population	35 CHD deaths/ 1,000 population
High Dietary Fat: 35% energy, chiefly unsaturated fat from plant oils	High Dietary Fat: 33% energy, chiefly saturated fat from animal sources

Fig. 2.1 Regional differences. *Source*: Seven counties study [2]

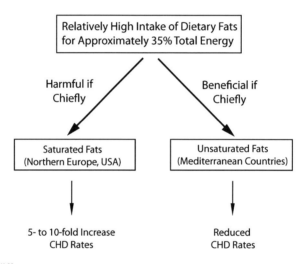

Fig. 2.2 Fat differences

associated with percentage of dietary energy obtained from unsaturated fatty acids [1, 2, 6]. This study advanced dietary knowledge of what is now one of the guiding principles for food choices in a MedDiet: different types of fats have very different health effects. Numerous additional studies have corroborated those differences in health effects among dietary fat sources [7–10]. An emphasis on high intake of healthy fats and low intake of unhealthy fats, as opposed to avoidance of all fats, is now considered an integral part of a MedDiet (Figs. 2.2 and 2.3).

The longest-lived populations in the Seven Countries study were from the heart of the Mediterranean regions where they consumed a diet that was primarily plant-based

Relationship of Saturated and Unsaturated Fats to Disease Risk

Amount of saturated fat ($^{\text{principally from}}_{\text{animal source}}$) consumed α disease risk

Amount of unsaturated fat ($^{\text{principally from}}_{\text{plant source}}$) consumed $1/\alpha$ disease risk

Fig. 2.3 Fat proportion to risk

Energy consumption in calories per day per person in 1961:

	Vegetable	Animal and Meat
Greece	2,450	470
Italy	2,460	600
Spain	2,270	445
United States	1,877	1,340

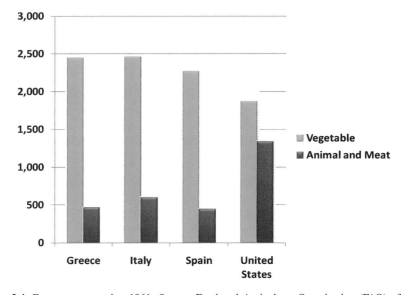

Fig. 2.4 Energy consumption 1961. *Source*: Food and Agriculture Organization (FAO) of the United Nations. Databank, Agriculture, Food Balance Sheet

and included abundant fruits, vegetables, nuts, seeds, unrefined cereals (grains), and infrequent meats and dairy. Nutrient sources in the Mediterranean countries and the United States during the 1960s are shown in Fig. 2.4.

Since this health-promoting dietary pattern was common in the Mediterranean regions, it was referred to as a "Mediterranean diet" with increasing frequency.

Ultimately, an attempt at a consensus for what its constituent nutrients were occurred at "The 1993 International Conference of the Diets of the Mediterranean." The results of this conference along with more contemporary published definitions can be combined to create an eight-point list summarizing the content of a MedDiet [2, 11–13]:

1. High intake of plant foods that are minimally processed and seasonally fresh. This includes fruits, vegetables, bread, unrefined cereals, beans, legumes, nuts, and seeds.
2. Olive oil as the primary source of dietary fat.
3. Moderate to low intake of dairy products, consumed chiefly as yogurt and cheese.
4. Moderate to low intake of poultry and low to very low intake of red meat and processed meat and meat products.
5. Daily wine in low to moderate amounts and generally with meals.
6. Less than four egg yolks per week.
7. Infrequent consumption of concentrated sweets.
8. Weekly or greater consumption of fish.

I have found it useful to define a MedDiet for patients by dividing its overall nutrient intake levels into high, moderate, and low categories. These are presented as follows:

1. High intake: Vegetables, fruits, nuts, legumes, whole grain carbohydrates, and plant oils (particularly olive and canola oils).
2. Moderate intake: Daily alcohol, fish at least once a week.
3. Low intake: Red meat and meat products, whole-fat dairy products, processed foods, simple and refined sugars, and egg yolks.

Additional methods to convey the foods within a MedDiet have taken the form of the traditional food pyramid. The Grand Hellenic Ministry of Greece created a Mediterranean Diet Pyramid that summarizes the foods and their quantity of consumption in an idealized MedDiet (Fig. 2.5).

The different qualitative descriptions outlined above can be useful as a general roadmap for patients who wish to understand and follow a MedDiet. A quantitative method for purposes of defining and analyzing a MedDiet in scientific studies also exists. This quantitative method allows researchers to assess how the extent of an individual's adherence to a MedDiet affects health outcomes, and it will be termed the Mediterranean diet adherence score (MedDiet-AS) in this book. It is calculated in the following fashion:

First, a researcher creates general food categories based on the major food groups in a MedDiet such as vegetables, whole grains, or healthy fats. Once the categories have been created, they are then designated as either favorable or unfavorable. The favorable food categories typically created are vegetables; fruits; nuts and legumes; whole grain products; high monounsaturated fatty acids to saturated fatty acids ratio; fish; and moderate alcohol. The unfavorable categories typically created are red and processed meat and whole-fat dairy

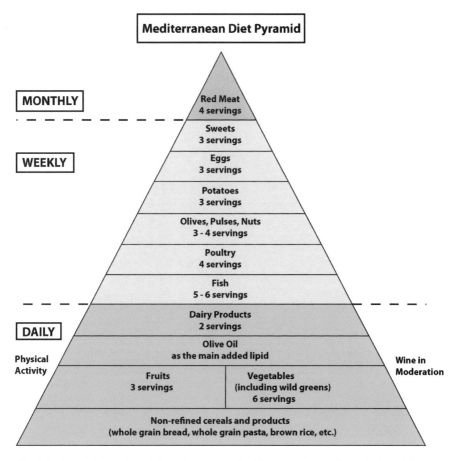

Fig. 2.5 Greek diet. Adapted from Supreme Scientific Health Council, Hellenic Ministry of Health

products. Next, the food categories are scored for individual participants. Favorable categories are assigned a value of one for a study participant who has consumed a quantity of the foods it contains at or above the gender-specific median consumption levels of those foods for all that study's participants. A score of zero is given if consumption is below the gender-specific median. An unfavorable food category is assigned a value of zero if the study participant being analyzed has consumed a quantity of those foods it contains at or above the gender-specific median or a value of one if below the median. The total MedDiet-AS scores will range from 0 points at lowest adherence to 7–13 points, depending on the number of separate categories created, at highest adherence (Fig. 2.6) [11, 13, 14, 15].

To help clarify the use of a MedDiet-AS, the two examples that follow can be helpful. The first example calculates a MedDiet-AS for a single, favorable food

Fig. 2.6 Scoring food

Calculating Mediterranean Diet Adherence Score

If food category is considered part of a Med-Diet:

Consumption levels above gender-specific median - add 1

Consumption levels below gender-specific median - add 0

If food category is not considered part of a Med-Diet:

Consumption levels above gender-specific median - add 0

Consumption levels below gender-specific median - add 1

category, such as vegetables. The second example calculates a MedDiet-AS for a single, unfavorable food category such as meat and meat products.

Example 1

If, in a population being studied, the gender-specific median consumption of vegetables is 30 servings per week, then individuals who average 30 or more servings per week would be given a value of one for the vegetable nutrient category. If an individual consumed an average of 29 or fewer servings per week, the score would be zero (Fig. 2.7).

Example 2

If, in a population being studied the gender-specific median consumption of meat and meat products is 5 servings per week, then individuals who average 5 or more servings per week would be given a value of zero for the meat and meat product nutrient category. If an individual consumed 4 or fewer servings per week, the score given would be one (Fig. 2.7).

To calculate the total MedDiet-AS, the process as shown in the two preceding examples is then applied to each of the nutrient categories in the study (Table 2.1, see Chap. 14). Individual authors may have chosen to combine some categories or to expand the number of categories resulting in a lower or higher total possible MedDiet-AS in their particular study.

In the next example, the calculation of a MedDiet-AS is applied to four individuals (Table 2.2). This further illustrates how, among different individuals, varying consumption levels within the nutrient categories will affect the MedDiet-AS.

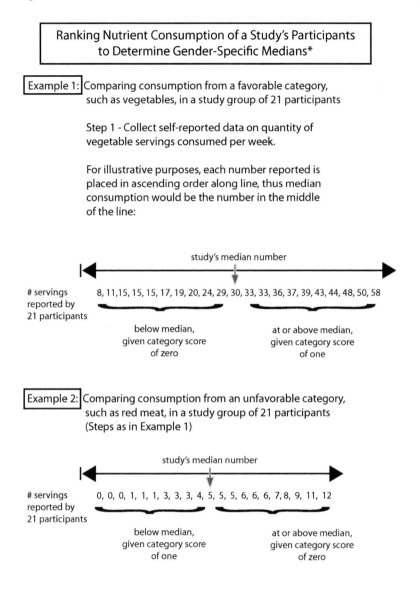

Ranking Nutrient Consumption of a Study's Participants
to Determine Gender-Specific Medians*

Example 1: Comparing consumption from a favorable category,
such as vegetables, in a study group of 21 participants

Step 1 - Collect self-reported data on quantity of
vegetable servings consumed per week.

For illustrative purposes, each number reported is
placed in ascending order along line, thus median
consumption would be the number in the middle
of the line:

study's median number

servings   8, 11,15, 15, 15, 17, 19, 20, 24, 29, 30, 33, 33, 36, 37, 39, 43, 44, 48, 50, 58
reported by
21 participants

below median,   at or above median,
given category score   given category score
of zero   of one

Example 2: Comparing consumption from an unfavorable category,
such as red meat, in a study group of 21 participants
(Steps as in Example 1)

study's median number

servings   0, 0, 0, 1, 1, 1, 3, 3, 3, 4, 5, 5, 5, 6, 6, 6, 7, 8, 9, 11, 12
reported by
21 participants

below median,   at or above median,
given category score   given category score
of one   of zero

* since this method compares subject's consumption level of a particular
nutrient only to that of his fellow subjects, the median would be specific
to that particular study's population

Fig. 2.7 Gender-specific median

Table 2.1 Calculating Mediterranean diet adherence score

Commonly used categories	Score given for consumption at or above gender-specific median	Score given for consumption below gender-specific median
Vegetables	1	0
Fruits	1	0
Legumes	1	0
Whole grains/cereals	1	0
Nuts and seeds	1	0
Monounsaturated fatty acid to saturated fatty acid ratio	1	0
Fish	1	0
Meat and meat products	0	1
Full-fat dairy products	0	1
Alcohol[a]	1[a]	0[a]
Optimal adherence total = 10		
Minimal adherence total = 0		

[a]For alcohol, score of 1 is given only if consumption falls within given, gender-specific parameters. Favorable parameters are:
For men: 10–50 g/day=1 (~1/2–2 drinks/day)
For women: 5–25 g/day=1 (~1/4–1 drink/day)

Table 2.2 Mediterranean diet adherence score for four individuals

Calculation of Mediterranean diet adherence score for four individuals

Categories	Individual #1 frequency[a]	Given points	Individual #2 frequency	Given points	Individual #3 frequency	Given points	Individual #4 frequency	Given points
Vegetables	Rare	0	Frequent	1	Frequent	1	Frequent	1
Fruits	Rare	0	Frequent	1	Frequent	1	Frequent	1
Legumes	Never	0	Rare	0	Frequent	1	Frequent	1
Whole grains/cereals	Never	0	Frequent	1	Rare	0	Frequent	1
Nuts and seeds	Rare nuts	0	Rare nuts	0	Rare nuts	0	Daily	1
MUFA/SFA	Frequent SFA	0	Frequent MUFA	1	Frequent SFA	0	Frequent MUFA	1
Fish	Never	0	Frequent	1	Rare	0	Frequent	1
Meat/meat products	Frequent	0	Rare	1	Frequent	0	Never	1
Full-fat dairy	Frequent	0	Rare	1	Rare	1	Never	1
Alcohol	Never	0	Heavy	0	Moderate	1	Moderate	1
Med-Di adherence score		0 of 10		7 of 10		5 of 10		10 of 10

[a]"Frequent" or "Daily" implies above gender-specific median levels. "Rare" or "Never" implies below gender-specific median levels

Table 2.3 shows patients dietary changes that can be made to optimize each category within a MedDiet.

The method for calculating a MedDiet-AS gives equal weight to the potential health effects of each nutrient category. The pattern as a whole is being evaluated,

Table 2.3 To increase MedDiet-AS

Changes in dietary pattern to maximize Mediterranean diet adherence score (AS)		
Nutrient consumption pattern that lowers Med-Di AS	Transform to increase Med-Di AS	Nutrient consumption pattern that raises Med-Di AS
Rare vegetables	→	Frequent, daily vegetables
Rare fruits	→	Frequent, daily fruits
Rare legumes	→	Frequent legumes
Rare whole grains	→	Frequent, daily whole grains
Rare nuts	→	Daily nuts
Frequent animal SFA, rare plant MUFA	→	Rare animal SFA, frequent plant MUFA
Rare fish	→	At least once weekly fish
Frequent meat and meat products	→	Rare meat and meat products
Frequent full-fat dairy	→	Rare dairy or only fat-free dairy
Either zero or heavy alcohol	→	Moderate alcohol

and no single food or category is given greater weight in the evaluation of health benefits. Additionally, the fact that a MedDiet-AS assesses total nutrient intake over a period of time means that an occasional unhealthy food choice will not adversely affect overall dietary benefit of a MedDiet. Knowing that their diet does not need to be perfect when following a MedDiet can be reassuring to patients and increase their long-term compliance.

References

1. Keys A, Parlin RW. Serum cholesterol response to changes in dietary lipids. Am J Clin Nutr. 1966;19:175–81.
2. Keys A, Menotti A, Karvonen MJ, Aravanis C, Blackburn H, Buzina R, et al. The diet and 15-year death rate in the seven countries study. Am J Epidemiol. 1986;124(6):903–15.
3. Nestle M. Mediterranean diets: historical and research overview. Am J Clin Nutr. 1995; 61(6 Suppl):1313S–20.
4. Tunstall-Pedoe H, Kuulasmaa K, Mähönen M, Tolonen H, Ruokokoski E, Amouyel P. Contribution of trends in survival and coronary-event rates to changes in coronary heart disease mortality: 10-year results from 37 WHO MONICA project populations. Monitoring trends and determinants in cardiovascular disease. Lancet. 1999;353(9164):1547–57.
5. Masiá R, Pena A, Marrugat J, Sala J, Vila J, Pavesi M, et al. High prevalence of cardiovascular risk factors in Gerona, Spain, a province with low myocardial infarction incidence. REGICOR investigators. J Epidemiol Community Health. 1998;52(11):707–15.
6. Keys A. Coronary heart disease–the global picture. Atherosclerosis. 1975;22(2):149–92.
7. Dwyer JT. Vegetarian eating patterns: science, values, and food choices–where do we go from here? Am J Clin Nutr. 1994;59(5 Suppl):1255S–62.
8. Kromhout D, Keys A, Aravanis C, Buzina R, Fidanza F, Giampaoli S, et al. Food consumption patterns in the 1960s in seven countries. Am J Clin Nutr. 1989;49(5):889–94.
9. Serra-Majem L, Ribas L, Lloveras G, Salleras L. Changing patterns of fat consumption in Spain. Eur J Clin Nutr. 1993;47 Suppl 1:S13–20.
10. U.S. Department of Agriculture. Center for Nutrition Policy and Promotion. Dietary guidelines for Americans. 2010. http://www.cnpp.usda.gov/dietaryguidelines.htm. Accessed 1 Jan 2011.

11. Trichopoulou A, Kouris-Blazos A, Wahlqvist ML, Gnardellis C, Lagiou P, Polychronopoulos E, et al. Diet and overall survival in elderly people. BMJ. 1995;311(7018):1457–60.
12. Martinez-Gonzalez MA, Estruch R. Mediterranean diet, antioxidants and cancer: the need for randomized trials. Eur J Cancer Prev. 2004;13(4):327–35.
13. Bach A, Serra-Majem L, Carrasco JL, Roman B, Ngo J, Bertomeu I, et al. The use of indexes evaluating the adherence to the Mediterranean diet in epidemiological studies: a review. Public Health Nutr. 2006;9(1A):132–46.
14. Martínez-González MA, Fernández-Jarne E, Serrano-Martínez M, Wright M, Gomez-Gracia E. Development of a short dietary intake questionnaire for the quantitative estimation of adherence to a cardioprotective Mediterranean diet. Eur J Clin Nutr. 2004;58(11):1550–2.
15. Sofi F, Cesari F, Abbate R, Gensini GF, Casini A. Adherence to Mediterranean diet and health status: meta-analysis. BMJ. 2008;337:a1344.

Part II
Effects on Diseases

Chapter 3
Mechanisms of Action and Effects on Diseases

Keywords Mediterranean diet • Mechanisms • Favorable effects • Morbidity • Mortality

A Mediterranean diet is associated with reduced risk for cardiovascular diseases, cancer, Alzheimer's disease, Parkinson's disease, rheumatoid arthritis and other arthritidies, asthma, atopy and allergic rhinitis, metabolic syndrome, and overall mortality. It has also demonstrated efficacy for obesity prevention and weight loss [1–3]. A framework to help patients conceptualize a MedDiet's benefits obtained from the favorable biological effects of its many healthy foods and its general avoidance of unhealthy foods is outlined in this chapter (Table 3.1).

An effective way to optimize patients' retention of the concept that what one eats directly affects the body's internal biology can be to sketch a diagram showing potential health consequences from prolonged exposure to either an optimal or a poor diet. Although Fig. 3.1 simplifies a tremendously complex process, it does demonstrate the key point that frequent poor food choices can overwhelm the body's intrinsic self-maintenance and repair mechanisms to result in clinical disease.

The clinical studies reviewed in this book have rated each nutrient category in a MedDiet equally so that the benefits reported have resulted from the entire dietary pattern's effects over a prolonged period of time. An important point is that just as one bad meal or poor food choice will not adversely affect long-term health outcomes, one good meal will not favorably compensate for an otherwise unhealthy diet. Occasionally eating foods or meals that are not perfect for health will not cause one to "fail" at a MedDiet. Conversely, adding one favorable food or occasional ideal meal to an otherwise poor diet will be of no significant benefit in preventing disease. Using these concepts, patients should be encouraged to adopt a long-term time horizon when thinking of the health effects of their diet and to understand that gradually, over time, consuming a preponderance of quality foods will reduce disease risk while the excess consumption of unfavorable foods will lead to increased risk.

E. Zacharias, *The Mediterranean Diet: A Clinician's Guide for Patient Care*,
DOI 10.1007/978-1-4614-3326-2_3, © Springer Science+Business Media, LLC 2012

Table 3.1 More favorable, less unfavorable

Conceptualization of simultaneous mechanisms of action of a med-Di		
Consumption of more favorable nutrients	→	Provides substrate for normal growth, metabolism, and repair in the tissues
Consumption of fewer, unfavorable nutrients	→	Provides less substrate for initiation and propagation of abnormal metabolism and disease in the tissues

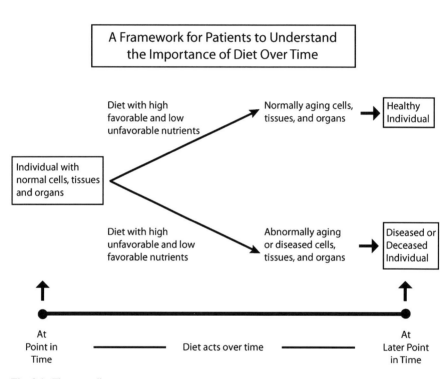

Fig. 3.1 Tissue to disease

It would be a nice problem if the worst dietary issue facing providers were that on occasion people with good diets briefly strayed from their healthy habits. Unfortunately, the reality is that a tremendous percentage of the population eats too much unhealthy food too often and eats too little healthy food too infrequently. As the Dietary Guidelines for Americans, 2010 has made clear, the recommended intake for many healthy foods in the U.S. is not close to being met, and the limit for many unhealthy foods is greatly exceeded [4]. Figure 3.2 graphically illustrates how far off we are from optimal targets.

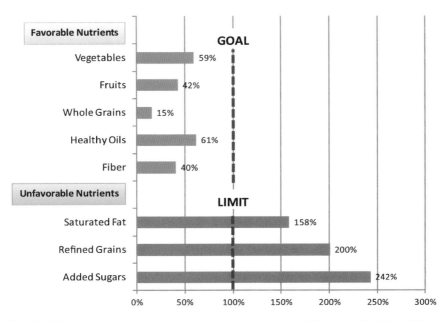

Fig. 3.2 How the typical American diet compares to recommended dietary intake. Adapted from US Dietary Guidelines for Americans, 2010 [4]

In the studies that follow, a MedDiet is demonstrated to be strongly associated with favorable health outcome (Fig. 3.3). Additionally, it may have a dose–response effect such that, for any Mediterranean Diet-adherence score (MedDiet-AS), the next greater MedDiet-AS results in a greater level of benefit. The studies selected for review have generally evaluated health outcome endpoints as opposed to biomarker endpoints. Although biomarkers may be important precursor changes indicating risk for development of disease, it is the actual effects of diet on disease that have the greatest clinical relevance. The editorial rigor of the major peer-reviewed scientific journals is considered adequate for presenting an article as evaluating study design and quality is beyond the scope and purposes of this book. Interested providers are encouraged to follow-up the references for further reading.

Summary of Important Studies Demonstrating Improved Survival with a Mediterranean Diet

An inverse relationship between a MedDiet and mortality has been demonstrated in numerous major studies [5–13].

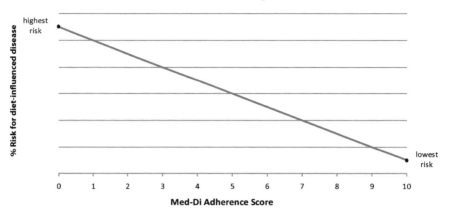

Fig. 3.3 Adherence and benefits

1995

The MedDiet-AS predicted survival in a cohort of nearly 200 adults over the age of 70. A single-point increase in a participant's MedDiet-AS was associated with a 17% reduction in relative risk for mortality, and a four-point increase in score was associated with a 50% reduction in mortality [14].

1997

A single-point increase in MedDiet-AS was associated with a 21% reduction in relative mortality risk over 6 years in a cohort study of more than 200 elderly patients [15].

1998

In the Lyon Diet Heart Study, patients with known coronary heart disease (CHD) were randomized to either a Mediterranean diet including fatty acid supplementation or a prudent, low-fat diet. The MedDiet patients showed a 56% reduced risk for death compared with those consuming the prudent, low-fat diet [16].

1999

A single-point increase in a MedDiet-AS was associated with a 17% reduction in overall mortality in a cohort study of more than 300 elderly Australians of both Greek and Anglo origin. The benefits were independent of a participant's ethnic heritage [17].

2000

A single-point increase in a MedDiet-AS was associated with a 31% reduction in mortality over 9 years in a cohort of more than 150 Spaniards aged 65–80 years [18].

2003

A two-point increase in MedDiet-AS was associated with a 25% reduction in mortality in a cohort of 22,000 Greek adults followed over 4 years. Authors of the study noted that of the ten separate categories they used to calculate a MedDiet-AS, no individual category could be demonstrated to confer stronger benefit than any others. Hence, they concluded that the overall dietary pattern was more important than any individual nutrient groups [11].

2004

Study participants with a total MedDiet-AS of four points or greater had a 22% reduction in mortality relative to those with a score less than four over a 10-year period in a longitudinal study of more than 2,300 elderly Europeans [9].

2005

A two-point increase in MedDiet-AS was associated with a 27% reduction in mortality rate in a group of more than 1,300 study participants with known CHD. No individual category comprising the scoring system was demonstrated to be superior in its beneficial effects [19].

2006

A two-point increase in a MedDiet-AS was associated with a 13% reduction in overall mortality over a 12-year period in a cohort of 42,000 Swedish women aged 40–49 years [20].

Leading nutritional and public health scientists modeled data showing that optimal adherence to a MedDiet, along with not smoking and regular physical activity would reduce our nation's burden of CHD by 80%, cerebrovascular accident (CVA) by 70%, and Type 2 diabetes (T2D) by 90% [21].

2007

Individuals with the highest adherence score (6–9 points) had a mortality reduction of 21% relative to those with the lowest score (0–3 points) in this cohort study of more than 375,000 American men and women [10].

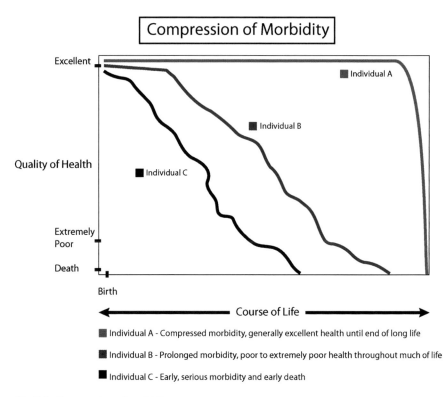

Fig. 3.4 Compression of morbidity

2008

A two-point increase in MedDiet-AS was associated with a 9% reduction in mortality in this meta-analysis of 12 prospective studies with a combined total of more than 1,500,000 subjects [1].

When I discuss the preceding trials with patients, I will often draw a diagram similar to that in Fig. 3.4 as an easy way to represent the concept of compression of morbidity to patients.

References

1. Sofi F, Cesari F, Abbate R, Gensini GF, Casini A. Adherence to Mediterranean diet and health status: meta-analysis. BMJ. 2008;337:a1344.
2. Serra-Majem L, Roman B, Estruch R. Scientific evidence of interventions using the Mediterranean diet: a systematic review. Nutr Rev. 2006;64(2 Pt 2):S27–47.
3. Martinez-Gonzalez MA, Bes-Rastrollo M, Serra-Majem L, Lairon D, Estruch R, Trichopoulou A. Mediterranean food pattern and the primary prevention of chronic disease: recent developments. Nutr Rev. 2009;67 Suppl 1:S111–6.
4. U.S. Department of Agriculture. Center for Nutrition Policy and Promotion. Dietary guidelines for Americans. 2010. http://www.cnpp.usda.gov/dietaryguidelines.htm. Accessed 1 Jan 2011.
5. Fidanza F, Alberti A, Lanti M, Menotti A. Mediterranean Adequacy Index: correlation with 25-year mortality from coronary heart disease in the Seven Countries Study. Nutr Metab Cardiovasc Dis. 2004;14(5):254–8.
6. Fung TT, Malik V, Rexrode KM, Manson JE, Willett WC, Hu FB. Sweetened beverage consumption and risk of coronary heart disease in women. Am J Clin Nutr. 2009;89(4):1037–42.
7. Fung TT, Rexrode KM, Mantzoros CS, Manson JE, Willett WC, Hu FB. Mediterranean diet and incidence of and mortality from coronary heart disease and stroke in women. Circulation. 2009;119(8):1093–100. Erratum in: Circulation. 2009;119(12):e379.
8. Harriss LR, English DR, Powles J, Giles GG, Tonkin AM, Hodge AM, Brazionis L, O'Dea K. Dietary patterns and cardiovascular mortality in the Melbourne Collaborative Cohort Study. Am J Clin Nutr. 2007;86(1):221–9.
9. Knoops KT, de Groot LC, Kromhout D, Perrin AE, Moreiras-Varela O, Menotti A, van Staveren WA. Mediterranean diet, lifestyle factors, and 10-year mortality in elderly European men and women: the HALE project. JAMA. 2004;292(12):1433–9.
10. Mitrou PN, Kipnis V, Thiébaut AC, Reedy J, Subar AF, Wirfält E, et al. Mediterranean dietary pattern and prediction of all-cause mortality in a US population: results from the NIH-AARP Diet and Health Study. Arch Intern Med. 2007;167(22):2461–8.
11. Trichopoulou A, Costacou T, Bamia C, Trichopoulos D. Adherence to a Mediterranean diet and survival in a Greek population. N Engl J Med. 2003;348(26):2599–608.
12. Trichopoulou A, Bamia C, Trichopoulos D. Anatomy of health effects of Mediterranean diet: Greek EPIC prospective cohort study. BMJ. 2009;338:b2337.
13. Waijers PM, Ocké MC, van Rossum CT, Peeters PH, Bamia C, Chloptsios Y, et al. Dietary patterns and survival in older Dutch women. Am J Clin Nutr. 2006;83(5):1170–6.
14. Trichopoulou A, Kouris-Blazos A, Wahlqvist ML, Gnardellis C, Lagiou P, Polychronopoulos E, et al. Diet and overall survival in elderly people. BMJ. 1995;311(7018):1457–60.
15. Osler M, Schroll M. Diet and mortality in a cohort of elderly people in a north European community. Int J Epidemiol. 1997;26(1):155–9.

16. de Lorgeril M, Salen P, Martin JL, Monjaud I, Boucher P, Mamelle N. Mediterranean dietary pattern in a randomized trial: prolonged survival and possible reduced cancer rate. Arch Intern Med. 1998;158(11):1181–7.
17. Kouris-Blazos A, Gnardellis C, Wahlqvist ML, Trichopoulos D, Lukito W, Trichopoulou A. Are the advantages of the Mediterranean diet transferable to other populations? A cohort study in Melbourne, Australia. Br J Nutr. 1999;82(1):57–61.
18. Lasheras C, Fernandez S, Patterson AM. Mediterranean diet and age with respect to overall survival in institutionalized, nonsmoking elderly people. Am J Clin Nutr. 2000;71(4):987–92.
19. Trichopoulou A, Bamia C, Trichopoulos D. Mediterranean diet and survival among patients with coronary heart disease in Greece. Arch Intern Med. 2005;165(8):929–35.
20. Lagiou P, Trichopoulos D, Sandin S, Lagiou A, Mucci L, Wolk A, Weiderpass E, Adami HO. Mediterranean dietary pattern and mortality among young women: a cohort study in Sweden. Br J Nutr. 2006;96(2):384–92.
21. Willett WC. The Mediterranean diet: science and practice. Public Health Nutr. 2006; 9(1A):105–10.

Chapter 4
Cardiovascular Diseases

Keywords Mediterranean diet • Cardiovascular disease • Atherosclerosis • Heart attack • Stroke • Saturated fatty acids • Monounsaturated fatty acids

Heart Attacks and Strokes

The observation in the 1950s and 1960s of a significantly lower incidence of cardiovascular disease (CVD) in the olive-growing, Mediterranean regions of Europe, compared with Northern Europe and the United States, was the initial reason the Mediterranean diet was studied. Since that time, a MedDiet has repeatedly demonstrated its ability to reduce the risk for CVD—the number one cause of mortality and years of life lost worldwide. Select statistics regarding CVD can educate patients about its importance:

- In the United States, 34% of all deaths are directly from CVD, and one third of these CVD deaths occur before the age of 75 years [1, 2].
- Every 25 s an American will have a coronary event [1, 2].
- Every 40 s an American will have a stroke [1, 2].
- Nearly half of all individuals with CVD are less than 60 years old [1].
- Women have a 500% greater risk of dying from CVD than from breast cancer [2].
- Over 17 million Americans currently have CHD [1–4].
- In 2007, there were nearly 80 million office visits in the the United States for CVD [2, 5, 6].
- Total direct and indirect costs of CVD for 2010 are estimated at $503 billion, making it the most costly of any disease in the United States [1].

E. Zacharias, *The Mediterranean Diet: A Clinician's Guide for Patient Care*,
DOI 10.1007/978-1-4614-3326-2_4, © Springer Science+Business Media, LLC 2012

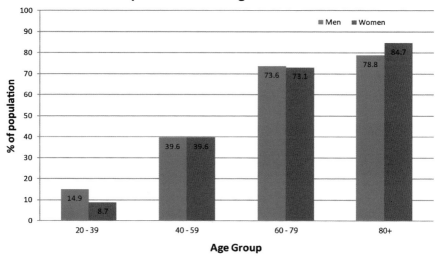

Fig. 4.1 Diagnosed cardiovascular disease. *Source*: NHANES: 2003-2006 [12]; NCHS [2]; NHLBI [13]

Although CVD is prevalent in the developed world, there are compelling data that it is largely a preventable disease. Modifiable risk factors have been shown to account for 85% or more of our nation's CVD, and, of these, diet and lifestyle choices are the most important components [7–10]. Unfortunately, Western societies are heading in the wrong direction in diet-related preventive measures. In the United States and much of the developed world, escalating rates of major CVD risk factors including obesity, type II diabetes (T2D), and hypertension (HTN), all directly attributable to diet, threaten to increase prevalence of CVD after 40 years of declining rates (Fig. 4.1) [11–13]. As health care providers, we should be at the forefront of this issue by seeking and implementing effective interventions for our patients of all ages to prevent initiation and reverse progression of atherosclerosis.

Looking at how well we do with preventing atherosclerosis in our youth can give insight into what society's future burden of CVD will be. Unfortunately, these data are discouraging, and they reveal that we have created a lifestyle and food environment causing atherosclerosis to occur at a high rate in our children (Fig. 4.2) [14]. In one study of more than 2,800 American youths under the age of 35 who died of external causes, autopsy was performed to evaluate for the presence of arterial fatty streaks, the earliest stage of atherosclerosis, and for the presence of advanced atherosclerosis. Fatty streaks were found in the right coronary arteries of approximately 58% of the study's 15- to 19-year-olds and in the aortas of nearly 100% of the 15- to 19-year-olds. Advanced atherosclerotic disease, present as raised arterial lesions, was present in the right coronary arteries of approximately 45% of the study's 30- to 34-year-olds and in the aortas of approximately 60% of the 30- to 34-year-olds [14].

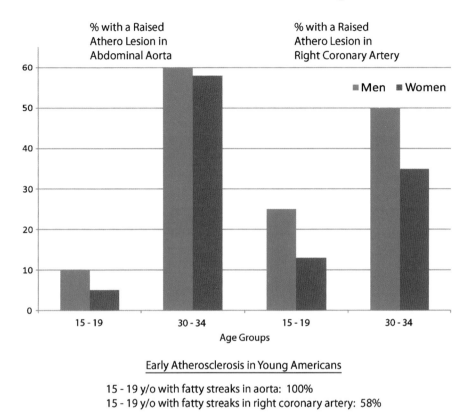

Fig. 4.2 Atherosclerosis in youth. Data from Strong et al. [14]

The importance of changing the atherogenic diets and lifestyles leading to high burdens of disease at such young ages is clear. Although children may not show clinical symptoms of atherosclerosis for many decades, the fact that the disease has already started in nearly all patients over age 15 in the United States means that, irrespective of age, individuals should be targeted for preventive lifestyle strategies. Chapter 16 offers constructive suggestions for healthy snacks and meals for busy parents and youths to substitute for many of today's common, unhealthy choices.

Atherosclerosis

When patients understand the basics of atherogenesis, I have found it increases their interest in and compliance with a preventive diet and lifestyle. The first point I make when explaining this complex process is that atherosclerosis actually occurs within the arterial walls, intramurally, and not attached to their inner surface, like grease

Where Atherosclerosis Occurs

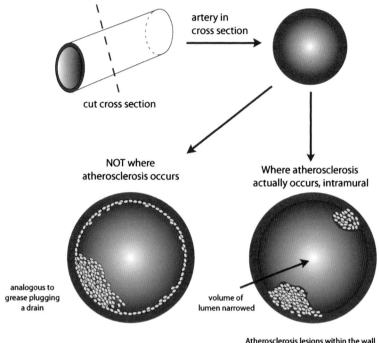

Fig. 4.3   Where atherosclerosis occurs

clogging a drain pipe, as is commonly taught. Understanding this location within the artery helps with further comprehension of the effects of different factors on atherogenesis. A simple way to show this location is to sketch an artery with inner and outer walls and illustrate where the atherosclerotic process occurs as shown in Fig. 4.3.

Once patients understand that atherosclerosis occurs intramurally, I explain that the process begins when the endothelial cells forming the protective inner lining of the vessel, called the intima, are exposed to pro-atherogenic factors such as those present in an unhealthy diet. These factors cause the intima to partially lose its integrity and allow the infiltration of low-density lipoproteins (LDL) and monocytes into the arterial wall. As this progresses, the infiltrated LDL becomes oxidized, monocytes phagocytize the oxidized LDL and transform into dysfunctional foam cells, and smooth muscle cells in the lesion start to proliferate. At this stage of atherogenesis, preventive medicine strategies can reverse the process, and the vessel's intrinsic self-repair mechanisms can return it toward a stable, non-diseased state. Understanding that atherosclerosis can be improved as well as worsened by diet may motivate patients to follow dietary advice (Fig. 4.4).

Atherosclerosis is Dynamic

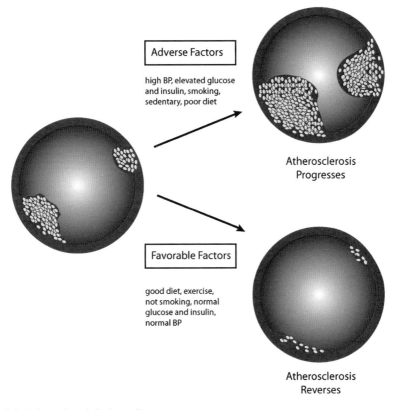

Adverse Factors

high BP, elevated glucose
and insulin, smoking,
sedentary, poor diet

Atherosclerosis
Progresses

Favorable Factors

good diet, exercise,
not smoking, normal
glucose and insulin,
normal BP

Atherosclerosis
Reverses

Fig. 4.4 Atherosclerosis is dynamic

With continued exposure of the vessel to disease-promoting factors, the atherosclerotic process advances, resulting in a highly active, inflamed, bulging lesion that protrudes into the lumen of the vessel. If this protrusion is large enough to cause obstruction of flow, then ischemic symptoms will be present in the area supplied by the vessel. At an advanced stage, the atherosclerotic progression may weaken the intima's endothelial cells to the point where they rupture and expose the lesion's highly thrombogenic internal components to the circulating blood. An acute thrombus may then form and obstruct the lumen, interrupting blood flow to the tissue the artery supplies. Clinical symptoms present based on what tissue the obstructed artery supplies (Fig. 4.5).

Atherosclerotic lesions progress or regress over time based partly on the intravascular milieu created by factors including blood pressure, blood glucose and insulin levels, cigarette smoking, exercise, and diet. Lifestyle interventions to address these factors are at least as effective, and significantly less expensive, for CVD prevention than medications [15]. For example, it has been shown that, per year of life

Progression from Normal Vessel to Atherosclerosis, to Event

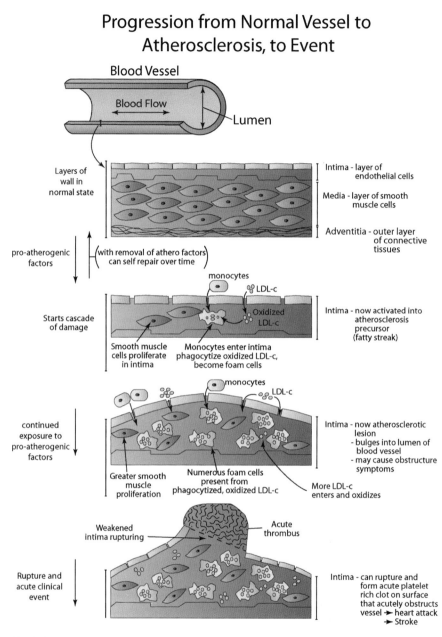

Fig. 4.5 Atherosclerosis

gained, costs run $10,000–$18,000 for statin drug therapy and as low as $20 for healthy eating [16] (Fig. 4.6). For individuals who require medications for treatment of risk factors, the benefits of diet and exercise are additive to those achieved from medications alone [17–19].

Mediterranean Diet as Anti-Atherogenic Diet

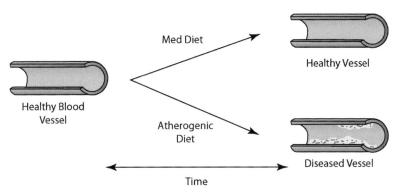

Fig. 4.6 MedDiet anti-atherosclerosis

Studies

CHD was the first disease process that a MedDiet was definitively shown to reduce. Due to its status as the number one cause of premature morbidity and mortality in the developed world, CHD has been the focus of the lion's share of MedDiet research studies. Reviewing the following studies with patients may help give them an understanding of the powerful effect of dietary choices in a MedDiet on CVD risks. A point to make is that the data presented may make a MedDiet seem too good to be true. However, the data are strong, consistent, and come from numerous different authors from different countries and include hundreds of thousands of unique patients. The totality of the published literature evaluating a MedDiet's effects on CVD has been so convincing that the 2010 Dietary Guidelines for Americans recommended a MedDiet as an effective dietary pattern for reducing the burden of CVD in the United States [20]. Although a MedDiet will not eliminate all CVD, its widespread adoption would be a tremendous public health advance.

1966

A diet low in saturated fat and high in polyunsaturated fat was described as key to reducing serum cholesterol and consequent CHD [21].

1980

The authors documented a nearly tenfold higher incidence of CHD in northern European regions when compared with the populations in the traditional olive-growing regions of Europe. The authors concluded that, although both populations had a similar consumption of total fat calories, those fats in the northern European population mostly comprised saturated fatty acids (SFA) of animal origin and those fats in the olive-growing region population mostly comprised unsaturated fatty acids of plant origin [22].

Author's note: This report from the famous "Seven Countries Trial" helped lead to the modern concept of a Mediterranean diet for health.

1986

Death rates from CHD were positively related to the percentage of SFA and negatively related to percentage of monounsaturated fatty acids (MUFA) in the diets of 11,500 initially healthy people who were followed over a period of 15 years [23].

1999

In study subjects with prior myocardial infarction, risk of death was reduced by approximately 70% in those randomized to dietary counseling on a Mediterranean-style diet supplemented with the polyunsaturated fatty acid alpha-linolenic acid and olive oil compared with those randomized to advice to consume a prudent diet [24].

Author's note: This was the final report from the famous "Lyon Heart Study" that furthered the understanding that fats of the monounsaturated- and polyunsaturated-fatty acid classes, when part of a total dietary pattern, are not only more healthy than saturated fats but can be more healthy than avoidance of fats altogether.

2002

In each of two study populations, one with and one without a history of CHD, every additional point in a MedDiet adherence score was associated with an 8% additional risk reduction for myocardial infarction [25].

In a study following more than 1,900 Greeks for 2 years, those who adopted a MedDiet had a 20% reduced risk of a coronary event [26].

2003

A higher adherence to a MedDiet was associated with a 33% reduced risk of death from CHD in this study of more than 22,000 health Greek adults [27].

In a study of more than 850 adults with diabetes type II (T2D), a MedDiet adherence score of 11 or greater on a 14 point scale was associated with a 56% reduced risk of peripheral artery disease compared to a score of less than 11 [28].

2004

More than 3,000 patients were placed into tertiles based on their MedDiet adherence score. Relative to the lowest tertile, those in the highest tertile had 20% lower C-reactive protein levels, 17% lower IL-6 levels, 15% lower homocysteine levels, and 6% lower fibrinogen levels. The authors concluded these reductions in inflammatory and coagulation markers might be one of the beneficial mechanisms of a MedDiet for CHD reduction [29].

This trial randomized patients with metabolic syndrome to either a MedDiet or a prudent, low-fat diet. At the end of the trial, the MedDiet group had significant improvement in CVD risk markers of C-reactive protein, IL-6, IL-7, IL-8, insulin resistance, and endothelial function. Additionally, the MedDiet group had more weight loss and a significant reduction in metabolic syndrome [30].

A Mediterranean Diet-adherence score (MedDiet-AS) of four or greater in an eight-category scale was associated with a 20% reduced risk of death from CHD in a cohort of 2,300 elderly Europeans when they were compared to individuals with a MedDiet-AS of less than four [31].

2005

Serum biological markers of atherosclerosis risk were significantly improved at 3 months in individuals randomized to a MedDiet vs. a prudent diet. The study authors predicted the level of improvement would translate into a 15% reduction in CVD [32].

Each one-point reduction (on an eight point scale) in MedDiet adherence score in a group of Israeli males was associated with an increase in risk of 20% for myocardial infarction, 60% for coronary artery by-pass surgery, 40% for angioplasty, and 30% for any CVD [33].

2006

A leading nutrition and public health expert determined that data on a MedDiet for disease prevention demonstrate that the United States could reduce its burden of CHD by 80%, stroke by 70%, and T2D by over 90% if its citizens uniformly adopted a MedDiet, never smoked, and maintained regular physical activity [10].

A MedDiet supplemented with either extra virgin olive oil or nuts was shown to improve CVD markers of plasma glucose levels, systolic blood pressure, and HDL-cholesterol ratio relative to a low-fat diet [34].

A higher adherence to a MedDiet pattern was associated with a significant reduction in risk for myocardial infarction in a case-control study of 340 participants [35].

A review of 35 experimental studies on MedDiet showed that it could stimulate favorable effects on lipoprotein levels, endothelial vasodilatation, insulin resistance, metabolic syndrome, and antioxidant capacity [36].

2007

In a study of more than 40,000 Australians, irrespective of country of birth, a MedDiet pattern was associated with a reduced risk for CVD mortality [37].

High adherence to a MedDiet, when compared to low adherence, was associated with a 20% decrease in all-cause mortality, a 22% decrease in CVD mortality, and a 12–17% decrease in cancer mortality in a study of more than 370,000 individuals [38].

2008

A two-point increase in a MedDiet adherence score was determined to result in a 9% reduction in mortality from CVD in this meta-analysis of 12 combined studies [39].

A dietary pattern of the same style of a MedDiet with increased intake of fruits and vegetables, legumes, fish, poultry, and whole grains showed a 28% relative risk reduction for CVD mortality in group of 77,000 female nurses. Additionally, higher intake of processed meats, red meat, refined grains, French fries, and sweets was associated with a 22% higher CV mortality [40]

2009

A group of 74,000 healthy women aged 38–63 years were divided into quintiles based upon MedDiet adherence scores. Those in the highest quintile, relative to the lowest quintile, had a 29% risk reduction for CHD, a 13% risk reduction for stroke, and a 39% risk reduction for mortality from CVD [41].

Highest MedDiet adherence was associated with a 40% reduced risk for CHD relative to lowest adherence, and each one-point increase in MedDiet adherence score was associated with a 6% reduced risk for CHD in a study of more than 41,000 individuals [42].

After a systematic literature review of more than 180 studies, the authors of this report concluded that the evidence for a MedDiet's ability to reduce CHD risk was strong, consistent, temporal, and coherent [43].

2010

The Dietary Guidelines for Americans, 2010 committee reviewed what they determined to be high-quality, major studies evaluating the health benefits of a MedDiet on CHD [27, 31, 37–39, 41, 43–46], and they concluded that a MedDiet pattern is beneficial for reducing the burden of CVD in the United States [20].

In this trial, a MedDiet was shown to reduce serum markers of inflammation, including C-reactive protein and LI-6. A low-fat diet was associated with an increase in these markers [47].

Overall

The preceding studies supply strong evidence that a MedDiet pattern with its emphasis on vegetables, fruits, whole-grain bread and cereals, nuts and seeds, healthy fats, fish, and moderate wine, and its infrequent whole-fat dairy and red meat and meat products is a highly effective approach to reducing patients' risks for the number one cause of death in the United States. The meal plans and recipes sections at the end of this book provide creative approaches to improve the diets of both our pediatric and adult patient populations in an effort to prevent or reverse the number one cause of death in the developed world.

References

1. American Heart Association (AHA). http://circ.ahajournals.org/content/123/4/e18.full.pdf. Accessed 27 May 2011.
2. National Center for Health Statistics (NCHS), 2011. http://www.cdc.gov/nchs/ Accessed 27 May 2011.
3. National Health Interview Survey (NHIS). http://www.cdc.gov/nchs/nhis.htm Accessed 27 May 2011.
4. Pleis JR, Lucas JW. Summary health statistics for U.S. adults: National Health Interview Survey, 2007. Vital Health Stat 10. 2009;240:1–159.
5. National Ambulatory Medical Care Survey (NAMCS). http://www.cdc.gov/nchs/ahcd.htm. Accessed 27 May 2011.
6. Hsiao CJ, Cherry DK, Beatty PC, Rechtsteiner EA. National Ambulatory Medical Care Survey: 2007 summary. Natl Health Stat Report. 2010;27:1–32.

7. Greenland P, Knoll MD, Stamler J, Neaton JD, Dyer AR, Garside DB, et al. Major risk factors as antecedents of fatal and nonfatal coronary heart disease events. JAMA. 2003;290(7):891–7.
8. Khot UN, Khot MB, Bajzer CT, Sapp SK, Ohman EM, Brener SJ, et al. Prevalence of conventional risk factors in patients with coronary heart disease. JAMA. 2003;290(7):898–904.
9. Daviglus ML, Lloyd-Jones DM, Pirzada A. Preventing cardiovascular disease in the 21st century: therapeutic and preventive implications of current evidence. Am J Cardiovasc Drugs. 2006;6(2):87–101.
10. Willett WC. The Mediterranean diet: science and practice. Public Health Nutr. 2006;9(1A): 105–10.
11. Lloyd-Jones D, Adams R, Carnethon M, De Simone G, Ferguson TB, Flegal K, et al. American heart association statistics committee and stroke statistics subcommittee. Heart disease and stroke statistics–2009 update: a report from the American Heart Association Statistics Committee and Stroke Statistics Subcommittee. Circulation. 2009;119(3):480–6.
12. Marriott BP, Olsho L, Hadden L, Connor P. Intake of added sugars and selected nutrients in the United States, national Health and Nutrition Examination Survey (NHANES) 2003-2006. Cr Rev Food Scie Nutr. 2010;50:228–58.
13. National Heart, Lung, and Blood Institute (NHLBI). http://www.nhlbi.nih.gov/health/public/heart/. Accessed 27 May 2011.
14. Strong JP, Malcom GT, McMahan CA, Tracy RE, Newman 3rd WP, Herderick EE, et al. Prevalence and extent of atherosclerosis in adolescents and young adults: implications for prevention from the Pathobiological Determinants of Atherosclerosis in Youth Study. JAMA. 1999;281(8):727–35.
15. Iestra JA, Kromhout D, van der Schouw YT, Grobbee DE, Boshuizen HC, van Staveren WA. Effect size estimates of lifestyle and dietary changes on all-cause mortality in coronary artery disease patients: a systematic review. Circulation. 2005;112(6):924–34.
16. Brunner E, Cohen D, Toon L. Cost effectiveness of cardiovascular disease prevention strategies: a perspective on EU food based dietary guidelines. Public Health Nutr. 2001;4(2B): 711–5.
17. Sdringola S, Nakagawa K, Nakagawa Y, Yusuf SW, Boccalandro F, Mullani N, et al. Combined intense lifestyle and pharmacologic lipid treatment further reduce coronary events and myocardial perfusion abnormalities compared with usual-care cholesterol-lowering drugs in coronary artery disease. JAm Coll Cardiol. 2003;41(2):263–72.
18. Chan SY, Mancini GB, Burns S, Johnson FF, Brozic AP, Kingsbury K, et al. Dietary measures and exercise training contribute to improvement of endothelial function and atherosclerosiseven in patients given intensive pharmacologic therapy. J Cardiopulm Rehabil. 2006;26(5): 288–93.
19. Daubenmier JJ, Weidner G, Sumner MD, Mendell N, Merritt-Worden T, Studley J, et al. The contribution of changes in diet, exercise, and stress management to changes in coronary risk in women and men in the multisite cardiac lifestyle intervention program. Ann Behav Med. 2007;33(1):57–68.
20. U.S. Department of Agriculture. Center for Nutrition Policy and Promotion. Dietary guidelines for Americans, 2010. http://www.cnpp.usda.gov/dietaryguidelines.htm. Accessed 1 Jan 2011.
21. Brown HB, Farrand ME. Pitfalls in constructing a fat-controlled diet. J Am Diet Assoc. 1966;49(4):303–8.
22. Keys Ancel. Seven countries: a multivariate analysis of death and coronary heart disease. Cambridge: Harvard University Press; 1980.
23. Keys A, Menotti A, Karvonen MJ, Aravanis C, Blackburn H, Buzina R, et al. The diet and 15-year death rate in the seven countries study. Am J Epidemiol. 1986;124(6):903–15.
24. de Lorgeril M, Salen P, Martin JL, Monjaud I, Delaye J, Mamelle N. Mediterranean diet, traditional risk factors, and the rate of cardiovascular complications after myocardial infarction: final report of the Lyon Diet Heart Study. Circulation. 1999;99(6):779–85.

25. Martínez-González MA, Fernández-Jarne E, Serrano-Martínez M, Marti A, Martinez JA, Martín-Moreno JM. Mediterranean diet and reduction in the risk of a first acute myocardial infarction: an operational healthy dietary score. Eur J Nutr. 2002;41(4):153–60.
26. Panagiotakos DB, Pitsavos C, Chrysohoou C, Stefanadis C, Toutouzas P. Risk stratification of coronary heart disease in Greece: final results from the CARDIO2000 Epidemiological Study. Prev Med. 2002;35(6):548–56.
27. Trichopoulou A, Costacou T, Bamia C, Trichopoulos D. Adherence to a Mediterranean diet and survival in a Greek population. N Engl J Med. 2003;348(26):2599–608.
28. Ciccarone E, Di Castelnuovo A, Salcuni M, Siani A, Giacco A, Donati MB, et al. Gendiabe Investigators. A high-score Mediterranean dietary pattern is associated with a reduced risk of peripheral arterial disease in Italian patients with Type 2 diabetes. J Thromb Haemost. 2003;1(8):1744–52.
29. Chrysohoou C, Panagiotakos DB, Pitsavos C, Das UN, Stefanadis C. Adherence to the Mediterranean diet attenuates inflammation and coagulation process in healthy adults: the ATTICA Study. J Am Coll Cardiol. 2004;44(1):152–8.
30. Esposito K, Marfella R, Ciotola M, Di Palo C, Giugliano F, Giugliano G, et al. Effect of a mediterranean-style diet on endothelial dysfunction and markers of vascular inflammation in the metabolic syndrome: a randomized trial. JAMA. 2004;292(12):1440–6.
31. Knoops KT, de Groot LC, Kromhout D, Perrin AE, Moreiras-Varela O, Menotti A, et al. Mediterranean diet, lifestyle factors, and 10-year mortality in elderly European men and women: the HALE project. JAMA. 2004;292(12):1433–9.
32. Vincent-Baudry S, Defoort C, Gerber M, Bernard MC, Verger P, Helal O, et al. The Medi-RIVAGE study: reduction of cardiovascular disease risk factors after a 3-mo intervention with a Mediterranean-type diet or a low-fat diet. Am J Clin Nutr. 2005;82(5):964–71.
33. Bilenko N, Fraser D, Vardi H, Shai I, Shahar DR. Mediterranean diet and cardiovascular diseases in an Israeli population. Prev Med. 2005;40(3):299–305.
34. Estruch R, Martínez-González MA, Corella D, Salas-Salvadó J, Ruiz-Gutiérrez V, Covas MI, et al.; PREDIMED Study Investigators. Effects of a Mediterranean-style diet on cardiovascular risk factors: a randomized trial. Ann Intern Med. 2006;145(1):1–11.
35. Martínez-González MA. The SUN cohort study (Seguimiento University of Navarra). Public Health Nutr. 2006;1A:127–31.
36. Serra-Majem L, Roman B, Estruch R. Scientific evidence of interventions using the Mediterranean diet: a systematic review. Nutr Rev. 2006;64(2 Pt 2):S27–47.
37. Harriss LR, English DR, Powles J, Giles GG, Tonkin AM, Hodge AM, et al. Dietary patterns and cardiovascular mortality in the Melbourne Collaborative Cohort Study. Am J Clin Nutr. 2007;86(1):221–9.
38. Mitrou PN, Kipnis V, Thiébaut AC, Reedy J, Subar AF, Wirfält E, et al. Mediterranean dietary pattern and prediction of all-cause mortality in a US population: results from the NIH-AARP Diet and Health Study. Arch Intern Med. 2007;167(22):2461–8.
39. Sofi F, Cesari F, Abbate R, Gensini GF, Casini A. Adherence to Mediterranean diet and health status: meta-analysis. BMJ. 2008;337:a1344.
40. Heidemann C, Schulze MB, Franco OH, van Dam RM, Mantzoros CS, Hu FB. Dietary patterns and risk of mortality from cardiovascular disease, cancer, and all causes in a prospective cohort of women. Circulation. 2008;118(3):230–7.
41. Fung TT, Rexrode KM, Mantzoros CS, Manson JE, Willett WC, Hu FB. Mediterranean diet and incidence of and mortality from coronary heart disease and stroke in women. Circulation. 2009;119(8):1093–100. Erratum in: Circulation. 2009;119(12):e379.
42. Buckland G, González CA, Agudo A, Vilardell M, Berenguer A, Amiano P, et al. Adherence to the Mediterranean diet and risk of coronary heart disease in the Spanish EPIC Cohort Study. Am J Epidemiol. 2009;170(12):1518–29.
43. Mente A, de Koning L, Shannon HS, Anand SS. A systematic review of the evidence supporting a causal link between dietary factors and coronary heart disease. Arch Intern Med. 2009;169(7):659–69.

44. Fidanza F, Alberti A, Lanti M, Menotti A. Mediterranean Adequacy Index: correlation with 25-year mortality from coronary heart disease in the Seven Countries Study. Nutr Metab Cardiovasc Dis. 2004;14(5):254–8.
45. Panagiotakos DB, Pitsavos C, Matalas AL, Chrysohoou C, Stefanadis C. Geographical influences on the association between adherence to the Mediterranean diet and the prevalence of acute coronary syndromes, in Greece: the CARDIO2000 study. Int J Cardiol. 2005;100(1): 135–42.
46. Panagiotakos D, Pitsavos C, Chrysohoou C, Palliou K, Lentzas I, Skoumas I, et al. Dietary patterns and 5-year incidence of cardiovascular disease: a multivariate analysis of the ATTICA study. Nutr Metab Cardiovasc Dis. 2009;19(4):253–63.
47. Estruch R. Anti-inflammatory effects of the Mediterranean diet: the experience of the PREDIMED study. Proc Nutr Soc. 2010;69(3):333–40.

Chapter 5
Alzheimer's Disease

Keywords Mediterranean diet • Alzheimer's disease • Monounsaturated fatty acids • Fish • Whole grains • Red wine

A MedDiet may prevent the development and slow the progression of Alzheimer's disease (AD). Although the data necessary to prove this benefit are incomplete, I think it is reasonable to advise patients that, thus far, the studies are promising.

Currently, there are more than five million Americans with AD, and its total annual costs are estimated to be $172 billion in direct care plus another $35 billion in annual lost productivity of employees who serve as caregivers for family members with AD [1, 2]. In the United States, the prevalence of Alzheimer's disease is 1–2% at age 65, 15% at age 75, and 40% at age 85 (Fig. 5.1). If nothing effective is done to reduce the risk for aging individuals, it is estimated that there will be a fivefold increase in the number of AD patients by the year 2050 [1] (Fig. 5.2).

In younger patients, I explain that making lifestyle changes today may pay future dividends when it comes to AD prevention and retention of cognition. I use Fig. 5.3 as a visual aid.

The main studies supporting recommendations for a MedDiet as a potential way to reduce risk for AD are summarized as follows:

2004

This literature review concluded that a high intake of monounsaturated fatty acids (MUFA), a regular consumption of fish, a regular intake of whole grain cereals, or a regular consumption of moderate amounts of red wine was associated with a reduced risk of developing AD. The authors noted a potential synergistic effect if an individual regularly consumed all three of these favorable foods, such as in a MedDiet. Additionally, the study reported that elderly populations in Japan, with

Fig. 5.1 Prevalence of AD.
Source: Alzheimer's
Association [1]

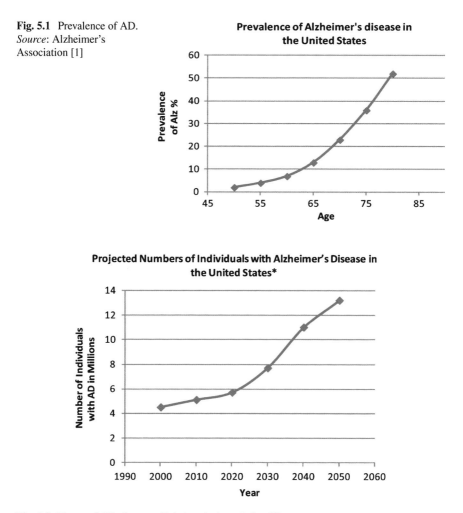

Fig. 5.2 Future of AD. *Source*: Alzheimer's Association [1]

a high intake of fish, have much lower rates of AD (<2%) in their native country than ethnic Japanese of similar age living in the United States (AD rate of 4.1%). The authors concluded that nutrition, lifestyle, and environment might play an important role in the development of AD [3].

2006

This prospective cohort study followed more than 2,200 nondemented, community-dwelling individuals in New York for 4 years. Their adherence to a MedDiet was scored zero to nine, with nine representing highest adherence, and individuals

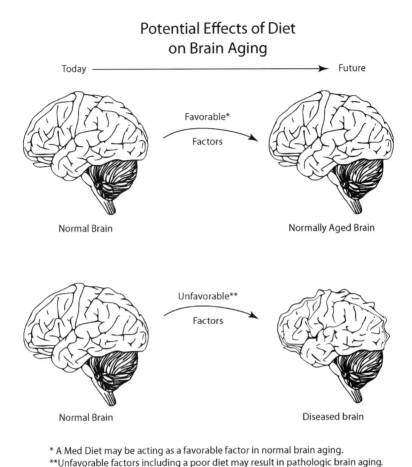

Potential Effects of Diet on Brain Aging

Today ————————————————————→ Future

Favorable*

Factors

Normal Brain   Normally Aged Brain

Unfavorable**

Factors

Normal Brain   Diseased brain

* A Med Diet may be acting as a favorable factor in normal brain aging.
**Unfavorable factors including a poor diet may result in pathologic brain aging.

Fig. 5.3 Potential diet effects

were grouped into tertiles based on their adherence scores. Over the course of the study, 250 individuals were diagnosed as developing AD. Individuals in the highest tertile of the adherence score (AS), most adherent, had the lowest risk for development of AD with a 40% risk reduction compared to those in the lowest tertile, least adherent [4].

This case-control study was nested within the cohort from the study noted previously. Traditional vascular variables including prior stroke, prior heart disease, diabetes, hypertension, and lipid levels were controlled for in study data analysis, and they did not affect the observed amount of AD risk reduction conferred by adherence to a MedDiet. In fact, after controlling for these vascular comorbidities, there was an even greater, 68%, risk reduction for AD relative to lowest adherence. The authors concluded a MedDiet might have beneficial effects on the brain in addition to effects on its vasculature that explain the risk reduction [5].

2007

This prospective cohort study followed nearly 200 community-based individuals in New York with a diagnosis of AD. Their adherence to a MedDiet was scored zero to nine, and individuals were grouped into tertiles based on their adherence scores. Those in the lowest tertile, reflecting lowest adherence to a Mediterranean diet, had the highest mortality. Those in the highest tertile, reflecting highest adherence, had the lowest mortality with a 73% risk reduction. The authors concluded this study demonstrated that, in addition to lowering risk for AD, a MedDiet lowers mortality in those who already have AD with a dose–response effect [6].

Although not designed to evaluate a MedDiet per se, this study examined the effects of key components of a MedDiet, frequent consumption of fruits and vegetables, fish, and omega-3 rich oils, and observed a reduction in dementia of 28–54% with this pattern compared to individuals with less frequent consumption of these foods [7].

2009

This prospective cohort study followed nearly 1,400 patients in New York who were diagnosed as cognitively normal at the start of the trial. Their adherence to a MedDiet was scored zero to nine, and individuals were grouped into tertiles based on their adherence scores. The authors concluded that a higher adherence to a MedDiet reduced risk both for development of mild cognitive impairment and for mild cognitive impairment progressing to Alzheimer's disease. Those in the highest tertile, reflecting highest adherence to a MedDiet, had a 48% risk reduction compared to those in the lowest tertile [8].

This prospective cohort study followed more than 1,400 nondemented, elderly French persons for an average of 2 years per individual during the study's 5-year period. Participants were assigned adherence to a MedDiet score. Individuals who remained dementia free based on results of the Mini-Mental State Examination (MMSE) were most likely to have the highest level of adherence to a Mediterranean diet. However, other cognitive screening tests used showed no similar relationships [9].

This prospective cohort study followed two cohorts with a combined total of nearly 1,900 patients. One cohort group was divided into tertiles based on adherence to MedDiet. The other cohort group was divided into tertiles based on amount of physical activity of its individuals. The study authors concluded that the combination of both higher physical activity and higher adherence to a MedDiet has an additive effect to lower risk for development of Alzheimer's disease by 35% [10].

2011

This trial evaluated association of adherence to a MedDiet or to the Healthy Eating Index-2005 and changes in cognitive function over time in a group of more than 3,700 individuals aged 65 years or greater. Over an average follow-up of 7 and 1½ years, individuals with higher adherence to a MedDiet showed significantly slower rates of cognitive decline than those with lower adherence. No association was noted with the Healthy Eating Index-2005 diet. The authors concluded that a MedDiet pattern might be helpful in slowing the rate of cognitive decline normally seen with aging [11].

References

1. Alzheimer's Association, facts and figures, 2010. http://www.alz.org/documents_custom/ report_alzfactsfigures2010.pdf. Accessed 27 May 2011.
2. Koppel R. Alzheimer's disease: the costs to U.S. businesses in 2002. Washington, DC: Alzheimer's Association; 2002.
3. Panza F, Solfrizzi V, Colacicco AM, D'Introno A, Capurso C, Torres F, Del Parigi A, Capurso S, Capurso A. Mediterranean diet and cognitive decline. Public Health Nutr. 2004;7(7):959–63.
4. Scarmeas N, Stern Y, Tang MX, Mayeux R, Luchsinger JA. Mediterranean diet and risk for Alzheimer's disease. Ann Neurol. 2006;59(6):912–21.
5. Scarmeas N, Stern Y, Mayeux R, Luchsinger JA. Mediterranean diet, Alzheimer disease, and vascular mediation. Arch Neurol. 2006;63(12):1709–17.
6. Scarmeas N, Luchsinger JA, Mayeux R, Stern Y. Mediterranean diet and Alzheimer disease mortality. Neurology. 2007;69(11):1084–93.
7. Barberger-Gateau P, Raffaitin C, Letenneur L, Berr C, Tzourio C, Dartigues JF, Alpérovitch A. Dietary patterns and risk of dementia: the Three-City cohort study. Neurology. 2007;69(20):1921–30.
8. Scarmeas N, Stern Y, Mayeux R, Manly JJ, Schupf N, Luchsinger JA. Mediterranean diet and mild cognitive impairment. Arch Neurol. 2009;66(2):216–25.
9. Féart C, Samieri C, Rondeau V, Amieva H, Portet F, Dartigues JF, et al. Adherence to a Mediterranean diet, cognitive decline, and risk of dementia. JAMA. 2009;302(6):638–48. Erratum in: JAMA. 2009;302(22):2436.
10. Scarmeas N, Luchsinger JA, Schupf N, Brickman AM, Cosentino S, Tang MX, Stern Y. Physical activity, diet, and risk of Alzheimer disease. JAMA. 2009;302(6):627–37.
11. Tangney CC, Kwasny MJ, Li H, Wilson RS, Evans DA, Morris MC. Adherence to a Mediterranean-type dietary pattern and cognitive decline in a community population. Am J Clin Nutr. 2011;93(3):601–7.

Chapter 6
Cancer

Keywords Mediterranean diet • Cancer • Mutagenesis • Promutagenic • Antimutagenic • Alpha-linolenic acid

Cancer is the most feared of all diseases in the United States [1]. It can be useful to explain to patients that while no known intervention, whether medication or diet and lifestyle, will reduce their risk for cancer to zero, they can optimize their risk through certain behaviors, including adopting a Mediterranean diet. The association between a reduction in cancer risk and a MedDiet was first reported in clinical trials designed primarily to evaluate cardiovascular disease end points. Once these studies revealed a potential cancer-reducing benefit, researchers subsequently designed trials to evaluate the effects of a MedDiet on the risk for developing or dying from cancer as primary endpoints.

Cancer is the second leading cause of death in the United States, responsible for 23% of all annual mortality [2]. The estimated annual costs for cancer health care are $228 billion in direct and indirect expenses [3]. The National Institutes of Health funds cancer research with an annual budget of more than $5 billion, making its research the most highly funded among all disease processes. Any intervention that reduces the risk of cancer would have major public health benefits and result in significant financial savings.

When I discuss a MedDiet's potentially protective role against cancer, I find sketching a simple office diagram showing how it can be conceptualized as promoting either pro- or antimutagenic processes proves to be a useful way to convey this point. I emphasize that anticancer properties of a MedDiet most likely arise from interactions among the numerous micronutrients consumed and from the fact that potentially promutagenic foods are consumed infrequently (Fig. 6.1). As with its effects on other diseases, it is the totality of the MedDiet, as opposed to a single nutrient, that provides its benefits against cancer.

E. Zacharias, *The Mediterranean Diet: A Clinician's Guide for Patient Care*, DOI 10.1007/978-1-4614-3326-2_6, © Springer Science+Business Media, LLC 2012

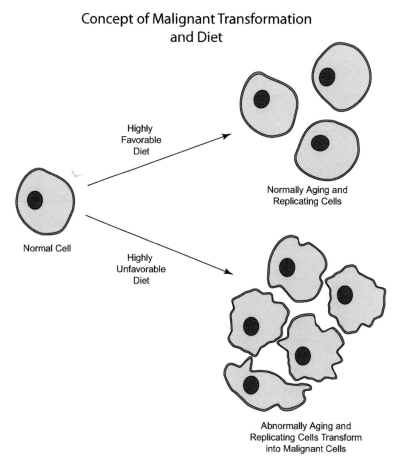

Fig. 6.1 Mutagenesis

The major studies that have evaluated the association between a MedDiet and cancer risk are presented chronologically as follows.

1998

In the "Lyon Diet Heart Study," individuals randomized to a MedDiet supplemented with alpha-linolenic acid (ALA) compared to individuals on a Step 1 AHA prudent diet showed a 61% reduced risk for development of cancer [4].

2003

Three case-control studies analyzing risks for upper respiratory and digestive tract cancers had their subjects' diets quantified with an eight-item MedDiet-adherence score (MedDiet-AS). A MedDiet-AS of six or greater, relative to a score of three or less, was associated with reduced cancer risk in the studies of 60, 74, and 77%, respectively [5].

2004

In the "HALE Project," among 2,300 healthy Europeans aged 70–90 there was a 10% reduction in cancer mortality risk with a MedDiet-AS of four or greater on an eight-point scale. Those with a score of four or greater who also exercised regularly, consumed moderate alcohol, and never smoked showed a 69% reduction in cancer mortality [6].

2006

In the "Nurses' Health Study" cohort, a nine-category MedDiet-AS was applied to dietary data of postmenopausal women. Relative to the lowest adherence quintile, women in the highest adherence quintile had a 21% reduced risk for estrogen receptor negative breast cancer [7].

In this trial, a ten-category MedDiet-AS was applied to dietary data of more than 42,000 women. A two-point increase in MedDiet-AS was associated with a 16% reduction in cancer mortality over 12 years in women aged 40–49 at time of study enrollment [8].

2007

In this prospective study of more than 380,000 individuals followed for 5 years, the authors concluded that, relative to low adherence, high adherence to a MedDiet was associated with a 17% reduced risk for cancer mortality in men and a 12% reduced risk in women [9].

Applying an eight category MedDiet-AS to participants aged 55–74 years in the "Prostate, Lung, Colorectal, and Ovarian Cancer Screening Trial," relative to a score of two or less, a MedDiet-AS of six or greater was associated with a 21% reduction in distal colorectal adenocarcinoma in men. No statistically significant difference was observed in women [10].

2008

In the Greek "EPIC" cohort study of more than 25,000 individuals, a two-point increase in a nine-category MedDiet-AS was associated with a 12% reduction in cancer incidence. The authors noted in their conclusion that the amount of risk reduction was greater than predicted for dietary components acting individually and, thus, the level of reduction might reflect synergistic interplay of the components of a MedDiet [11].

A nine-category MedDiet-AS was applied to more than 490,000 participants in the "NIH-AARP Diet and Health Study," and, compared to the lowest quintile, the highest quintile was associated with a relative risk reduction of 28% in men and 11% in women for colon cancer [12].

In the "Four Corners Breast Cancer Study" a MedDiet was associated with an odds ratio of 0.76 for development of cancer while a defined Western diet and Prudent diet were associated with odds ratios of 1.32 and 1.42, respectively [13].

2009

In the 485,000 participant "EPIC" cohort study, high adherence to a MedDiet was associated with a 33% reduction in risk for gastric adenocarcinoma relative to low adherence [14].

In a study of more than 1,200 Asian-American women, on a ten-category MedDiet-AS, a score of eight or greater was associated with a 35% reduction in breast cancer relative to a score of three or less. Additionally, women deemed to be high consumers of a "Western meat and starch diet" had an elevated odds ratio of 2.19 for breast cancer [15].

2010

After a review of 12 major epidemiological studies that had evaluated a MedDiet as an entire food pattern, the authors of this paper concluded that a MedDiet has a "probable" protective role in cancer reduction. The authors noted the potential public health importance of the anticancer properties of a MedDiet [16].

References

1. MetLife Foundation. What America thinks: MetLife Foundation Alzheimer's survey. Harris Interactive; February 2011.
2. Centers for Disease Control. National Center for Health Statistics (NCHS), 2011. http://www.cdc.gov/nchs/. Accessed 27 May 2011.
3. American Cancer Society. Cancer facts and figures, 2011. www.cancer.org/research/cancerfactsfigures/index. Accessed 27 May 2011.
4. de Lorgeril M, Renaud S, Mamelle N, Salen P, Martin JL, Monjaud I, et al. Mediterranean alpha-linolenic acid-rich diet in secondary prevention of coronary heart disease. Lancet. 1994;343(8911):1454–9.
5. Bosetti C, Gallus S, Trichopoulou A, Talamini R, Franceschi S, Negri E, et al. Influence of the Mediterranean diet on the risk of cancers of the upper aerodigestive tract. Cancer Epidemiol Biomarkers Prev. 2003;12(10):1091–4.
6. Knoops KT, de Groot LC, Kromhout D, Perrin AE, Moreiras-Varela O, Menotti A, et al. Mediterranean diet, lifestyle factors, and 10-year mortality in elderly European men and women: the HALE project. JAMA. 2004;292(12):1433–9.
7. Fung TT, Hu FB, McCullough ML, Newby PK, Willett WC, Holmes MD. Diet quality is associated with the risk of estrogen receptor-negative breast cancer in postmenopausal women. J Nutr. 2006;136(2):466–72.
8. Lagiou P, Trichopoulos D, Sandin S, Lagiou A, Mucci L, Wolk A, et al. Mediterranean dietary pattern and mortality among young women: a cohort study in Sweden. Br J Nutr. 2006;96(2):384–92.
9. Mitrou PN, Kipnis V, Thiébaut AC, Reedy J, Subar AF, Wirfält E, et al. Mediterranean dietary pattern and prediction of all-cause mortality in a US population: results from the NIH-AARP Diet and Health Study. Arch Intern Med. 2007;167(22):2461–8.
10. Dixon LB, Subar AF, Peters U, Weissfeld JL, Bresalier RS, Risch A, et al. Adherence to the USDA Food Guide, DASH Eating Plan, and Mediterranean dietary pattern reduces risk of colorectal adenoma. J Nutr. 2007;137(11):2443–50.
11. Benetou V, Trichopoulou A, Orfanos P, Naska A, Lagiou P, Boffetta P, et al. Conformity to traditional Mediterranean diet and cancer incidence: the Greek EPIC cohort. Br J Cancer. 2008;99(1):191–5.
12. Reedy J, Mitrou PN, Krebs-Smith SM, Wirfält E, Flood A, Kipnis V, et al. Index-based dietary patterns and risk of colorectal cancer: the NIH-AARP Diet and Health Study. Am J Epidemiol. 2008;168(1):38–48.
13. Murtaugh MA, Sweeney C, Giuliano AR, Herrick JS, Hines L, Byers T, et al. Diet patterns and breast cancer risk in Hispanic and non-Hispanic white women: the Four-Corners Breast Cancer Study. Am J Clin Nutr. 2008;87(4):978–84.
14. Buckland G, Agudo A, Luján L, Jakszyn P, Bueno-de-Mesquita HB, Palli D, et al. Adherence to a Mediterranean diet and risk of gastric adenocarcinoma within the European Prospective Investigation into Cancer and Nutrition (EPIC) cohort study. Am J Clin Nutr. 2010;91(2):381–90.
15. Wu AH, Yu MC, Tseng CC, Stanczyk FZ, Pike MC. Dietary patterns and breast cancer risk in Asian American women. Am J Clin Nutr. 2009;89(4):1145–54.
16. Verberne L, Bach-Faig A, Buckland G, Serra-Majem L. Association between the Mediterranean diet and cancer risk: a review of observational studies. Nutr Cancer. 2010;62(7):860–70.

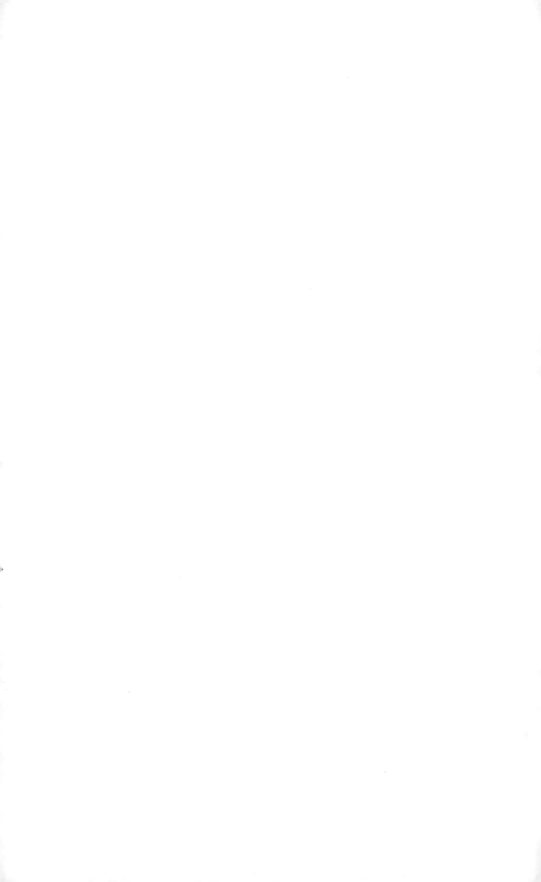

Chapter 7
Arthritis, Allergies, and Immunologic Disorders

Keywords Mediterranean diet • Arthritis • Asthma • Allergy • Immunologic • Anti-inflammatory

Arthritis, allergies, and other immunologic conditions are common, and it is not unusual for patients to ask for advice on an "anti-inflammatory" diet to help prevent or control them. As will be apparent from several clinical trials that are reviewed here, a MedDiet may be considered to serve as an "anti-inflammatory diet" to help prevent or control these conditions.

In explaining how diet affects immunologic conditions, I like the technique of sketching a quick office diagram as a visual aid (see Fig. 7.1). To acquire an immunologically mediated disorder, one must first have a certain baseline genetic predisposition that was then subject to further environmental factors. Over time, these factors, such as diet, stress, and infection, may "activate" the genetic predisposition and lead to the development of clinical disease. This outcome is not inevitable, and some individuals with a genetic predisposition never develop disease. Additionally, if disease is already present, environmental factors further affect the course and symptoms through multiple actions.

The chronologic summary of important trials that have evaluated a MedDiet for effects on immunologic conditions that follows provides information for further discussions and reading:

2003

In this trial, patients with rheumatoid arthritis were randomized to either a MedDiet or to no dietary intervention. At 12-week follow-up, those patients randomized to a MedDiet experienced significant improvement in pain, function, morning stiffness, and vitality as well as overall symptoms "compared to 1 year earlier." Those patients who continued a standard diet showed no improvement in any of the measures [1].

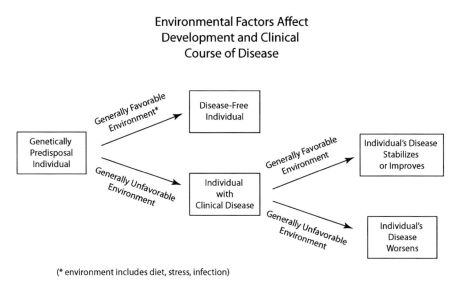

Fig. 7.1 Factors on genetics

2007

Authors of this study calculated a 12 category MedDiet adherence score (AS) for children aged 7–18 years using food questionnaires completed by their parents. It was concluded that a high MedDiet-AS was associated with a significant reduction in a child's risk for developing allergic rhinitis, wheezing, and atopy [2].

In this study, 130 women aged 30–70 years with rheumatoid arthritis were randomized to either attend cooking and education classes encouraging a MedDiet or to receive written educational materials on healthful eating. At 6 months follow-up, the MedDiet group showed significant improvement in global assessment, pain score, and early morning stiffness compared to the control group [3].

2008

This study calculated the MedDiet-AS of 174 adult asthmatics. The authors concluded that a high adherence to a MedDiet reduced the risk for noncontrolled asthma by 78% compared to low adherence [4].

In this study, a MedDiet-AS was calculated for the diet of pregnant women to see its effects on childhood allergic conditions. The authors concluded that, compared to a low MedDiet-AS, a high MedDiet-AS during pregnancy reduced the risk for the birth child at 6.5 years follow-up of having a persistent wheeze by 78%, an atopic wheeze by 70%, and atopy by 45% [5].

This trial demonstrated that, in 6- to 7-year-old children, adherence to a MedDiet was associated with reduced risk of asthma, wheezing, rhinitis, sneezing, and itchy-watery eyes. The authors concluded a MedDiet has a possible protective effect on asthma and allergic rhinitis [6].

Authors of this study sought to determine if a MedDiet might be protective against wheezing in preschool-aged children. After determining children's adherence to a MedDiet, it was concluded that a MedDiet is protective for current wheezing in preschoolers [7].

2010

The authors of this study sought to assess the effects of dietary factors on asthma and allergies. After analysis of dietary and symptom data from over 50,000 children, they concluded that adherence to a MedDiet, and particularly fruits, vegetables, and fish, was associated with protection against wheezing and asthma in childhood [8].

References

1. Sköldstam L, Hagfors L, Johansson G. An experimental study of a Mediterranean diet intervention for patients with rheumatoid arthritis. Ann Rheum Dis. 2003;62(3):208–14.
2. Chatzi L, Apostolaki G, Bibakis I, Skypala I, Bibaki-Liakou V, Tzanakis N, Kogevinas M, Cullinan P. Protective effect of fruits, vegetables and the Mediterranean diet on asthma and allergies among children in Crete. Thorax. 2007;62(8):677–83.
3. McKellar G, Morrison E, McEntegart A, Hampson R, Tierney A, Mackle G, et al. A pilot study of a Mediterranean-type diet intervention in female patients with rheumatoid arthritis living in areas of social deprivation in Glasgow. Ann Rheum Dis. 2007;66(9):1239–43.
4. Barros R, Moreira A, Fonseca J, de Oliveira JF, Delgado L, Castel-Branco MG, Haahtela T, Lopes C, Moreira P. Adherence to the Mediterranean diet and fresh fruit intake are associated with improved asthma control. Allergy. 2008;63(7):917–23.
5. Chatzi L, Torrent M, Romieu I, Garcia-Esteban R, Ferrer C, Vioque J, Kogevinas M, Sunyer J. Mediterranean diet in pregnancy is protective for wheeze and atopy in childhood. Thorax. 2008;63(6):507–13.
6. de Batlle J, Garcia-Aymerich J, Barraza-Villarreal A, Antó JM, Romieu I. Mediterranean diet is associated with reduced asthma and rhinitis in Mexican children. Allergy. 2008;63(10): 1310–6.
7. Castro-Rodriguez JA, Garcia-Marcos L, Alfonseda Rojas JD, Valverde-Molina J, Sanchez-Solis M. Mediterranean diet as a protective factor for wheezing in preschool children. J Pediatr. 2008;152(6):823–8, 828.e1–2.
8. Nagel G, Weinmayr G, Kleiner A, Garcia-Marcos L, Strachan DP, ISAAC Phase Two Study Group. Effect of diet on asthma and allergic sensitisation in the International Study on Allergies and Asthma in Childhood (ISAAC) Phase Two. Thorax. 2010;65(6):516–22.

Chapter 8
Diabetes and Metabolic Syndrome

Keywords Mediterranean diet • Metabolic syndrome • Blood glucose • HDL cholesterol • Triglycerides • Blood pressure • Waist circumference • Diabetes • Type 2 diabetes

The beneficial effects of a MedDiet on the prevention and reversal of diabetes and metabolic syndrome likely arise both from a MedDiet's actions on the intrinsic pathophysiology of the diseases themselves as well as from its effects on their major risk factors: overweight and obesity.

Metabolic syndrome is discussed first since, for all intents and purposes, it is a "prediabetic" state.

Metabolic syndrome was first defined as a specific entity in 2001 to identify patients at high risk for developing cardiovascular disease (CVD) and type 2 diabetes (T2D). The presence of metabolic syndrome increases a patient's risk for CVD by 65% and for T2D by 300% [1]. At least three of the following criteria must be present in a patient to meet the formal diagnosis for metabolic syndrome: elevated fasting blood glucose, low HDL cholesterol, elevated triglycerides, increased waist circumference, and elevated blood pressure. Currently, one-third of American adults meet the diagnostic criteria for metabolic syndrome [2]. This number will almost certainly continue to increase without a radical change in our current dietary pattern, and immediate intervention is warranted.

More than 50 major studies evaluating the effects of a MedDiet on metabolic syndrome have been published. A comprehensive review of these studies and trials with a combined total of more than 530,000 patients was published in 2011 and is an authoritative summary. Its authors determined that the body of literature demonstrates that adherence to a MedDiet has favorable effects on the individual metabolic syndrome components of blood glucose levels, HDL-c, triglycerides, blood pressure, and waist circumference, and reduces metabolic syndrome by an average of 31% when controlled for weight loss. The reduction in metabolic syndrome is even greater in patients who simultaneously lost weight [3].

Diabetes

Diabetes is a major risk factor for heart disease, strokes, blindness, kidney disease, neuropathy, and lower limb amputation. In recent estimates, nearly 10% of the adult population in the United States has diabetes, and this rate increases to 27% in individuals aged 65 years or greater [4–6]. The incidence of T2D, characterized by insulin resistance and relative insulin deficiency, has doubled in the past 30 years paralleling the rise in obesity [7]. Indeed, each 1 kg increase in body weight has been shown to increase risk for T2D by 7.3% [8]. The direct and indirect costs of diabetes are estimated at $174 billion annually and will almost certainly increase over the coming decades [9]. Stemming the rising tide of diabetes is a public health imperative. A MedDiet has been demonstrated to be effective in preventing and reversing both T2D and its precursor, metabolic syndrome, independent of its benefits on weight loss.

Recent studies evaluating the effect of a MedDiet on diabetes are summarized here.

2008

A trial using a nine category MedDiet-AS reported an 83% reduction in relative risk for development of T2D with a high adherence (score greater than 6) compared to a low adherence (score of 2 or less). Additionally, this trial reported that each two-point increase in MedDiet-AS reduced risk for diabetes by 35% [10].

2009

In this trial, overweight patients with a new diagnosis of T2D were randomized to either a MedDiet or a low-fat diet. At 4-year follow-up, the MedDiet group had greater weight loss and greater improvements in glycemic control and coronary risk measures than the low-fat diet group [11].

2011

In this trial, a MedDiet reduced the incidence of diabetes by 52% over a 4-year follow-up compared to a low-fat control diet. The authors noted that this favorable effect occurred without caloric restriction [12].

References

1. Expert Panel on Detection, Evaluation, and Treatment of High Blood Cholesterol in Adults. Executive Summary of the Third Report of the National Cholesterol Education Program (NCEP) Expert Panel on Detection, Evaluation, and Treatment of High Blood Cholesterol in Adults (Adult Treatment Panel III). JAMA. 2001;285(19):2486–97.
2. Ervin RB. Prevalence of metabolic syndrome among adults 20 years of age and over, by sex, age, race and ethnicity, and body mass index: United States, 2003–2006. Natl Health Stat Report. 2009;13:1–7.
3. Kastorini CM, Milionis HJ, Esposito K, Giugliano D, Goudevenos JA, Panagiotakos DB. The effect of Mediterranean diet on metabolic syndrome and its components: a meta-analysis of 50 studies and 534,906 individuals. J Am Coll Cardiol. 2011;57(11):1299–313.
4. National Institute of Diabetes and Digestive and Kidney Diseases. National diabetes statistics fact sheet: general information and national estimates on diabetes in the United States, 2005. Bethesda, MD: US Department of Health and Human Services, National Institutes of Health; 2005.
5. American Heart Association (AHA). http://circ.ahajournals.org/content/123/4/e18.full.pdf. Accessed 27 May 2011.
6. American Diabetes Association. http://www.diabetes.org/news-research/research/?loc=DropDownNR-research. Accessed 23 Nov 2011.
7. Fox CS, Pencina MJ, Meigs JB, Vasan RS, Levitzky YS, D'Agostino Sr RB. Trends in the incidence of type 2 diabetes mellitus from the 1970s to the 1990s: the Framingham Heart Study. Circulation. 2006;113(25):2914–8.
8. Koh-Banerjee P, Wang Y, Hu FB, Spiegelman D, Willett WC, Rimm EB. Changes in body weight and body fat distribution as risk factors for clinical diabetes in US men. Am J Epidemiol. 2004;159(12):1150–9.
9. National Institute of Diabetes and Digestive and Kidney Diseases. National diabetes statistics fact sheet: general information and national estimates on diabetes in the United States, 2008. Bethesda, MD: US Department of Health and Human Services, National Institutes of Health; 2008.
10. Martínez-González MA, de la Fuente-Arrillaga C, Nunez-Cordoba JM, Basterra-Gortari FJ, Beunza JJ, Vazquez Z, et al. Adherence to Mediterranean diet and risk of developing diabetes: prospective cohort study. BMJ. 2008;336(7657):1348–51.
11. Esposito K, Maiorino MI, Ciotola M, Di Palo C, Scognamiglio P, Gicchino M, et al. Effects of a Mediterranean-style diet on the need for antihyperglycemic drug therapy in patients with newly diagnosed type 2 diabetes: a randomized trial. Ann Intern Med. 2009;151(5):306–14.
12. Salas-Salvadó J, Bulló M, Babio N, Martínez-González MÁ, Ibarrola-Jurado N, Basora J, et al.; PREDIMED Study Investigators. Reduction in the incidence of type 2 diabetes with the Mediterranean diet: results of the PREDIMED-Reus nutrition intervention randomized trial. Diabetes Care. 2011;34(1):14–9.

Part III
Weight Loss and Obesity

Chapter 9
Weight, Obesity

Keywords Mediterranean diet • Weight • Overweight • Obesity • Body mass index

> The DGAC, 2010 considers the obesity epidemic to be the single greatest threat to public health this century (Dietary Guidelines for Americans Committee (DGAC) [1]).

This sober assessment from one of the most important health expert panels in the United States highlights the need for effective interventions to reduce overweight and obesity. Although most people prefer their appearance when they are leaner, the primary reason to address overweight and obesity with patients is that these are major health risks that markedly increase coronary heart disease, stroke, heart failure, diabetes, hypertension, sleep apnea, asthma, cancer, arthritis, and mortality, as well as contributing to multiple adverse psychological and social consequences [2–5]. In this chapter, our current problem of overweight and obesity is outlined, characteristics of a successful weight loss diet are discussed, and practical ideas for the use of a MedDiet for weight control are offered. The quantity of information presented is greater than can be shared with patients in a single office visit so this chapter may be used as a clinical reference to refer to as necessary. This chapter may also be offered to patients as a guide for independent follow-up reading on an effective, science-based strategy for weight loss.

One of the interesting challenges for a provider addressing obesity with patients is that the status of the provider's weight is obvious. Patients may view lean providers as not fully understanding the challenges of losing and keeping weight off since they are obviously not overweight. Irrespective of how diligently a provider may be working at personal weight control, patients may assume that one who is lean comes by that weight easily. Overweight or obese providers face the potential challenge of a credibility issue. If what they are sharing is actually important for health and the strategies being offered are effective, then their obvious lack of personal success may be discrediting. Providers may want to have a preencounter explanation prepared to address this paradox, such as:

E. Zacharias, *The Mediterranean Diet: A Clinician's Guide for Patient Care*, DOI 10.1007/978-1-4614-3326-2_9, © Springer Science+Business Media, LLC 2012

These strategies are proven to work, but as a human myself, I do not always do my best either.

Or

I have to sustain a diligent approach every day with these strategies to continue at my current weight.

It is important to address these concerns as indicated and then move forward to focus on the patient's care rather than dwelling on the provider's weight status.

A synopsis of the personal anecdote I share to show patients I understand what is required to lose and keep weight off follows:

I have lost 50 lb since graduating from medical school in 1993. I have kept that weight off without any appreciable regain for 18 years and counting, and I plan on never gaining it back. This has been accomplished by following a MedDiet and by increasing my daily activity level. In my experience, the foods in a MedDiet keep me feeling full and satisfied longer than the less healthy foods I used to consume to excess. I must remain conscientious to avoid overeating, to remain active, and to weigh myself frequently to ensure I am staying on track. As it is for anyone else, my success with weight control requires a lifelong effort.

Epidemiology, Definitions, Importance

It is important to know the common definitions and categorizations when discussing weight control. Overweight and obesity are categories that reflect the presence and extent of excess body fat. In the clinical and research setting, the most commonly used number to quantify a patient's weight is the body mass index (BMI), which is calculated in Fig. 9.1.

In children, a pediatric BMI for age growth chart is used. The categories for weight based on these measurements in adults and children are illustrated in Tables 9.1 and 9.2, and Figs. 9.2 and 9.3.

It should be noted that in very muscular individuals, providers must use clinical judgment when BMI is used. In this situation, waist circumference (measured at widest girth above the hip girdle and below the rib cage) may be used as an adjunct. A measurement of 40 or greater inches in men or 35 or greater inches in women is predictive of excess body fat and obesity.

The Extent of Our Problem

As a population, the United States is the most obese among all developed nations [6]. Data show that this epidemic developed rapidly with obesity nearly tripling since the 1970s in both adults and children [7, 8] (Fig. 9.4). In 1990, no states had obesity levels of greater than 15%, but by 2005 all 50 states had levels of over 15% obesity and only four states were under 20%. By 2009, only one state remained

Fig. 9.1 Calculation of body mass index (BMI)

Calculation of Body Mass index (BMI)

$$BMI = \frac{Weight\ (kg)}{Height\ Squared\ (m^2)} \quad or \quad \frac{Weight\ (pounds) \times 703}{Height\ Squared\ (inches^2)}$$

Table 9.1 Weight categorization by age

Weight classifications for BMI		
	Adults (BMI) kg/m^2	Pediatric ages (BMI for age in percentiles)
Underweight	<18.5	<5th
Healthy weight	18.5–24.9	5–84.9
Overweight	25–29.9	85–94.9
Obese	≥30	>95
Extreme obesity	≥40	

under 20% obesity, Colorado, and 33 states had reached levels of over 25% [6]. These trends reflect a nearly universal worsening of our problem.

Adults

At present, the number of Americans who are overweight or obese far exceeds the number at normal weight. Approximately 66% of the US adult population are overweight or obese, and about 33% overall are obese [6]. As noted, the increase in obesity rate has also occurred very rapidly, and this is surely related to recent dietary and lifestyle changes as it is implausible to speculate Americans have undergone a genetic transformation over 3 decades (Figs. 9.5 and 9.6).

Kids

The rapidly rising levels of overweight and obesity in children are perhaps even more troubling than those in adults (Figs. 9.7 and 9.8). Among all children, currently 32% are overweight or obese and 16% overall are obese, an increase of over 300% since 1970 when just 5% of all children were obese [6, 9]. Overweight adolescents have a 70% chance of becoming overweight adults [10, 11]. The obesity epidemic has become so pervasive in adolescents and young adults that, as one measure of effects on our society, over 25% of Americans age 17–24 are too overweight to qualify for military service [12]. The health effects of this are worrisome. In a long-term study with 50 years of follow-up, obese adolescents had a 230% higher all-cause mortality than their lean peers [13]. In addition to having the

Table 9.2 Adult BMI table

	Normal						Overweight					Obese										Extreme obesity														
BMI	19	20	21	22	23	24	25	26	27	28	29	30	31	32	33	34	35	36	37	38	39	40	41	42	43	44	45	46	47	48	49	50	51	52	53	54
Height (inches)	Body weight (pounds)																																			
58	91	96	100	105	110	115	119	124	129	134	138	143	148	153	158	162	167	172	177	181	186	191	196	201	205	210	215	220	224	229	234	239	244	248	253	258
59	94	99	104	109	114	119	124	128	133	138	143	148	153	158	163	168	173	178	183	188	193	198	203	208	212	217	222	227	232	237	242	247	252	257	262	267
60	97	102	107	112	118	123	128	133	138	143	148	153	158	163	168	174	179	184	189	194	199	204	209	215	220	225	230	235	240	245	250	255	261	266	271	276
61	100	106	111	116	122	127	132	137	143	148	153	158	164	169	174	180	185	190	195	201	206	211	217	222	227	232	238	243	248	254	259	264	269	275	280	285
62	104	109	115	120	126	131	136	142	147	153	158	164	169	175	180	186	191	196	202	207	213	218	224	229	235	240	246	251	256	262	267	273	278	284	289	295
63	107	113	118	124	130	135	141	146	152	157	163	169	175	180	186	191	197	203	208	214	220	225	231	237	242	248	254	259	265	270	278	282	287	293	299	304
64	110	116	122	128	134	140	145	151	157	163	169	174	180	186	192	197	204	209	215	221	227	232	238	244	250	256	262	267	273	279	285	291	296	302	308	314
65	114	120	126	132	138	144	150	156	162	168	174	180	186	192	198	204	210	216	222	228	234	240	246	252	258	264	270	276	282	288	294	300	306	312	318	324
66	118	124	130	136	142	148	155	161	167	173	179	186	192	198	204	210	216	223	229	235	241	247	253	260	266	272	278	284	291	297	303	309	315	322	328	334
67	121	127	134	140	146	153	159	166	172	178	185	191	198	204	211	217	223	230	236	242	249	255	261	268	274	280	287	293	299	306	312	319	325	331	338	344
68	125	131	138	144	151	158	164	171	177	184	190	197	203	210	216	223	230	236	243	249	256	262	269	276	282	289	295	302	308	315	322	328	335	341	348	354
69	128	135	142	149	155	162	169	176	182	189	196	203	209	216	223	230	236	243	250	257	263	270	277	284	291	297	304	311	318	324	331	338	345	351	358	365
70	132	139	146	153	160	167	174	181	188	195	202	209	216	222	229	236	243	250	257	264	271	278	285	292	299	306	313	320	327	334	341	348	355	362	369	376
71	136	143	150	157	165	172	179	186	193	200	208	215	222	229	236	243	250	257	265	272	279	286	293	301	308	315	322	329	338	343	351	358	365	372	379	386
72	140	147	154	162	169	177	184	191	199	206	213	221	228	235	242	250	258	265	272	279	287	294	302	309	316	324	331	338	346	353	361	368	375	383	390	397
73	144	151	159	166	174	182	189	197	204	212	219	227	235	242	250	257	265	272	280	288	295	302	310	318	325	333	340	348	355	363	371	378	386	393	401	408
74	148	155	163	171	179	186	194	202	210	218	225	233	241	249	256	264	272	280	287	295	303	311	319	326	334	342	350	358	365	373	381	389	396	404	412	420
75	152	160	168	176	184	192	200	208	216	224	232	240	248	256	264	272	279	287	295	303	311	319	327	335	343	351	359	367	375	383	391	399	407	415	423	431
76	156	164	172	180	189	197	205	213	221	230	238	246	254	263	271	279	287	295	304	312	320	328	336	344	353	361	369	377	385	394	402	410	418	426	435	443

Source: http://www.nhlbi.nih.gov/guidelines/obesity/bmi_tbl.htm

CDC Growth Charts: United States

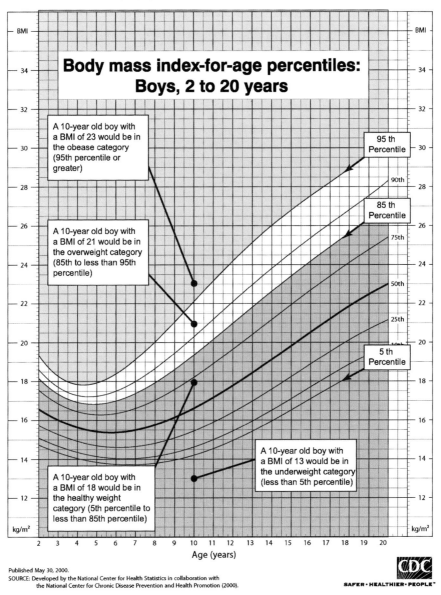

Body mass index-for-age percentiles: Boys, 2 to 20 years

A 10-year old boy with a BMI of 23 would be in the obease category (95th percentile or greater)

A 10-year old boy with a BMI of 21 would be in the overweight category (85th to less than 95th percentile)

A 10-year old boy with a BMI of 18 would be in the healthy weight category (5th percentile to less than 85th percentile)

A 10-year old boy with a BMI of 13 would be in the underweight category (less than 5th percentile)

95 th Percentile

85 th Percentile

5 th Percentile

90th
75th
50th
25th

Age (years)

Published May 30, 2000.
SOURCE: Developed by the National Center for Health Statistics in collaboration with the National Center for Chronic Disease Prevention and Health Promotion (2000).

SAFER · HEALTHIER · PEOPLE

Fig. 9.2 Boys BMI chart. Modified from Centers for Disease Control (CDC) growth charts. http://www.cdc.gov/growthcharts/data/set1clinical/Cj41cs023c.pdf

CDC Growth Charts: United States

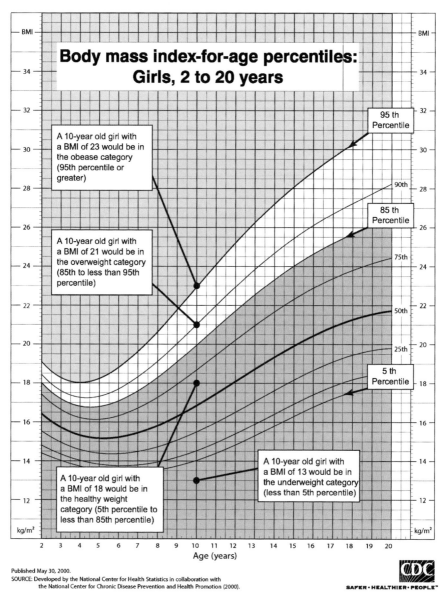

Body mass index-for-age percentiles: Girls, 2 to 20 years

A 10-year old girl with a BMI of 23 would be in the obease category (95th percentile or greater)

A 10-year old girl with a BMI of 21 would be in the overweight category (85th to less than 95th percentile)

95 th Percentile

85 th Percentile

90th

75th

50th

25th

5 th Percentile

A 10-year old girl with a BMI of 13 would be in the underweight category (less than 5th percentile)

A 10-year old girl with a BMI of 18 would be in the healthy weight category (5th percentile to less than 85th percentile)

Age (years)

Published May 30, 2000.
SOURCE: Developed by the National Center for Health Statistics in collaboration with the National Center for Chronic Disease Prevention and Health Promotion (2000).

Fig. 9.3 Girls BMI chart. Modified from Centers for Disease Control (CDC) growth charts. http://hp2010.nhlbihin.net/portion/servingcard7.pdf

Obesity Has Rapidly Risen

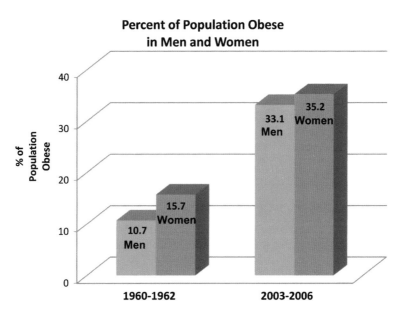

Fig. 9.4 Obesity rising. *Source*: CDC NCHS [6]

Fig. 9.5 Percentage of obese adults in 1960–1962 compared to 2003–2006

numerous health risks noted for adults, a major concern for overweight and obese children are the adverse social, educational, and psychological effects associated with excess weight during childhood and adolescence [14].

The reality is we are failing miserably at controlling the obesity epidemic in the United States. Without drastic changes in our current obesogenic American diet and lifestyle, by 2030 over 86% of Americans will be overweight or obese, and 51% overall will be obese [15]. Among concerns associated with this coming public health crisis are its enormous costs. Currently, medical care for obese adults is estimated to cost $1,500 more per year than care for normal weight individuals.

Fig. 9.6 Pie chart showing
percentage of healthy weight
compared to overweight
or obese adults in the United
States

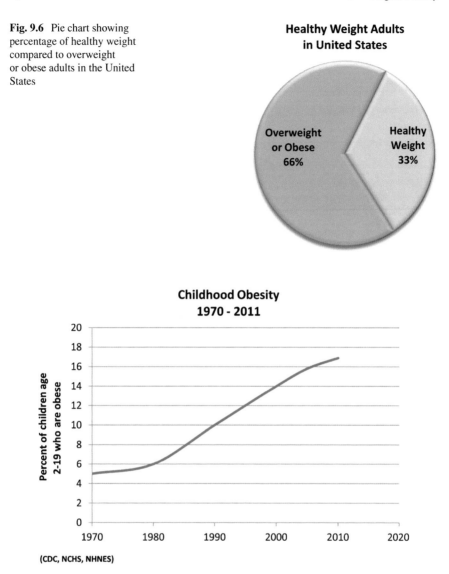

**Healthy Weight Adults
in United States**

Overweight
or Obese
66%

Healthy
Weight
33%

**Childhood Obesity
1970 - 2011**

(CDC, NCHS, NHNES)

Fig. 9.7 Obesity rise in children from 1970 to 2011. *Source*: CDC NCHS [6], NHANES[18]

This adds approximately $150 billion per year to America's health care costs [16]. The excess costs alone of overweight and obesity are predicted to reach more than $900 billion by 2030 if current trends continue [15]. It seems obvious that in a nation with limited financial resources, the favorable fiscal implications of any reduction in overweight and obesity would be a call to action for our nation's leaders. As a country, we must demand better of ourselves or the costs in increased morbidity and mortality and health care dollars will be catastrophic in the near future.

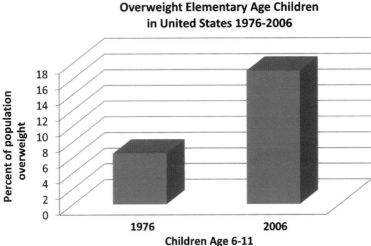

Fig. 9.8 Elementary-age children who are overweight

Science, Calorie Balance

A scientific explanation of how the balance between calories consumed and calories burned results in one's body weight can be a good place to start with patients when discussing weight loss and control. I like to start with a simple statement of fact: based on the first law of thermodynamics, one's body weight is a reflection of his or her energy balance (Fig. 9.9). When in positive energy balance, the intake of energy as food calories is greater than the amount of energy the body burns, and the excess energy is stored as body fat and weight increases. In negative energy balance, the intake of energy as food calories is less than the amount of energy the body burns, and the stored energy in the body, chiefly body fat, is mobilized for energy and thus weight decreases. When an individual is in neutral energy balance, consumption of total calories equals the calories the body requires and weight remains stable. Thus, to lose weight, I explain that a patient must eat less, exercise more, or do both to enter a negative energy balance. It is an absolute and inviolable law of thermodynamics that they cannot possibly gain body weight (other than, of course, water weight) without consuming more calories than they burn and that they absolutely must lose weight if they consume fewer calories than they burn.

Energy balance is affected by variables that may differ significantly among individuals, including physical activity, body size, age, gender, and basal metabolic rate. Additionally, basal metabolic rate may auto-adjust to a lower level in cases of caloric reduction. Due to these factors, at isocaloric consumption, one individual may be in negative energy balance and another in positive energy balance. Patients may indeed be correct when they believe that, relative to others, they consume very

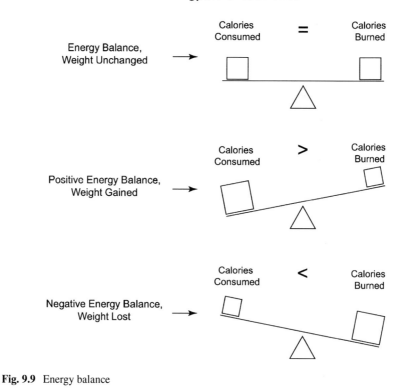

Fig. 9.9 Energy balance

little but still do not lose weight. However, if they achieve a negative energy balance they will still lose weight. Following body weight over time is the best way to assess energy balance in an individual patient.

Food Environment

Academic researchers have identified several changes over recent decades that account for the dramatic increase in overweight and obesity in the United States. Foremost, the cause of the obesity epidemic has been an increase in daily caloric consumption without a corresponding increase in physical activity. Since 1970, the average daily caloric intake has increased approximately 22% in women and 10% in men [17, 18]. Changes in our food environment, defined as all aspects of acquiring and consuming food, have favored excess caloric consumption. These changes have occurred in calories consumed, portion sizes, locations of meals consumed, energy density of foods, and locations at which foods are available for purchase [19–25]. Aspects of the food environment and how to improve them will now be discussed in more detail.

Portion Size

The first aspect of the current American food environment to discuss is portion size: the overall volume of food served at any time during a meal. There is a strong and positive relationship between portion size and body weight reported in numerous trials and reviews, and portion size has increased significantly since the 1970s [1, 17, 26–28]. Individuals with unrestricted, ad libitum access to food will consume more calories at a meal when they have larger portion sizes on their plates or in their bowls versus smaller portion sizes [29–31]. This same phenomenon is noted with snacking with larger portion sizes of the snacks resulting in greater caloric consumption [30, 32]. Patients should be cognizant that the modern phenomenon of large portion sizes for meals and snacks can easily sabotage their best efforts at weight loss.

Another issue is that as portion sizes have increased so have the sizes of plates and bowls that are used to serve food. Something as simple as using smaller sized plates and bowls has been shown to decrease portion size and total caloric consumption in ad libitum food access situations and to result in weight loss [17, 33]. Two figures follow. The first graphically illustrates to what extent our portion sizes have recently increased and the amount of extra physical activity that must be performed after each meal just to maintain caloric balance when consuming larger sized servings (Fig. 9.10). The second is a National Institute of Health guide to healthy portion sizes (Fig. 9.11) [34].

There are several suggestions providers can offer to patients for reducing portion size in common scenarios. Essentially, the goal of these is to cue the brain that smaller portion sizes equate to a full meal. When at a restaurant, patients can split their entrée with a dining companion or can ask that half of the meal is put into a "to-go bag" before food is brought to the table. A half of the modern, larger restaurant portions quickly seems normal. A similar strategy can be employed at quick-serve restaurants where a full-sized meal, such as a sandwich or burrito, is split with a friend or half of a meal is brought home for consumption at another mealtime or to share.

When making a meal at home one has more control of the food environment, but paying attention to portion size is necessary to help avoid excess calories. As noted, smaller sized plates and bowls are shown to reduce total caloric consumption so using smaller bowls and 9- to 10-in. plates will make the serving of reasonable-sized portions "fill the plate." Also, to optimize time efficiency, one can prepare enough food for multiple meals at one time and put the food not immediately served into storage containers and into the refrigerator or freezer before sitting down to eat.

a

Calorie + Portion Increase
Common Foods Over 20 Years :
Portion Distortion

Calorie Increase

Common Food	1990	2010	Activity + Duration Just to Balance Change
Bagel (+) 210 cal.	3" Diameter 140 Calories	6" Diameter 350 Calories	Rake Leaves* 50 Minutes
Cheeseburger (+) 257 cal.	333 Calories	590 Calories	Lift Weights* 1 Hour 30 Minutes
Spaghetti with Meatballs (+) 525 cal.	500 Calories 1 Cup Pasta, 3 Small Meatballs	1025 Calories 2 Cups Pasta, 3 Large Meatballs	House Cleaning* for 2 Hours 35 Minutes
French Fries (+) 400 cal.	2.4 oz. 210 Calories	6.9 oz. 610 Calories	Walk Leisurely** 1 Hour 10 Minutes
Soda (+) 165 cal.	6.5 oz. 85 Calories	20 oz. 250 Calories	Gardening** 35 Minutes
Turkey Sandwich (+) 500 cal.	320 Calories	800 Calories	Bike** 1 Hour 25 Minutes
Coffee (+) 305 cal.	8 oz. Coffee with Whole Milk + Sugar 45 Calories	16 oz. Mocha Coffee with Steamed Whole Milk and Mocha Syrup 350 Calories	Walk* 1 Hour 20 Minutes

* 130 lbs person
** 160 lbs person

Fig. 9.10 (**a**, **b**) Portion distortion. *Source*: US Department of Health and Human Services, NHLBI. http://hp2010.nhlbihin.net/oei_ss/PD1/slide1.htm

b

Calorie + Portion Increase
Common Foods Over 20 Years:
Portion Distortion

Calorie Increase			Activity + Duration
Common Food	1990	2010	Just to Balance Change
Muffin (+) 290 cal.	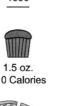 1.5 oz. 210 Calories	4 oz. 500 Calories	Vacuum* 1 Hour 30 Minutes
Pepperoni Pizza (+) 350 cal.	500 Calories	850 Calories	Golf while Walking and Carrying Clubs** 1 Hour
Chicken Caesar Salad (+) 400 cal.	390 Calories 1.5 Cup	790 Calories 3.5 Cups	Walk Dog** 1 Hours 20 Minutes
Popcorn (+) 360 cal.	5 Cups 270 Calories	11 Cups 630 Calories	Water Aerobics** 1 Hour 15 Minutes
Cheese Cake (+) 380 cal.	3 oz. 260 Calories	7 oz. 640 Calories	Play Tennis* 55 Minutes
Chocolate Chip Cookie (+) 220 cal.	55 Calories 1.5 Inch Diameter	275 Calories 3.5 Inch Diameter	Wash Car* 1 Hour 15 Minutes
Chicken Stir Fry (+) 305 cal.	435 Calories 2 Cups	865 Calories 4.5 Cups	Aerobic Dance* 1 Hour 5 Minutes

* 130 lbs person
** 160 lbs person

Fig 9.10 (continued)

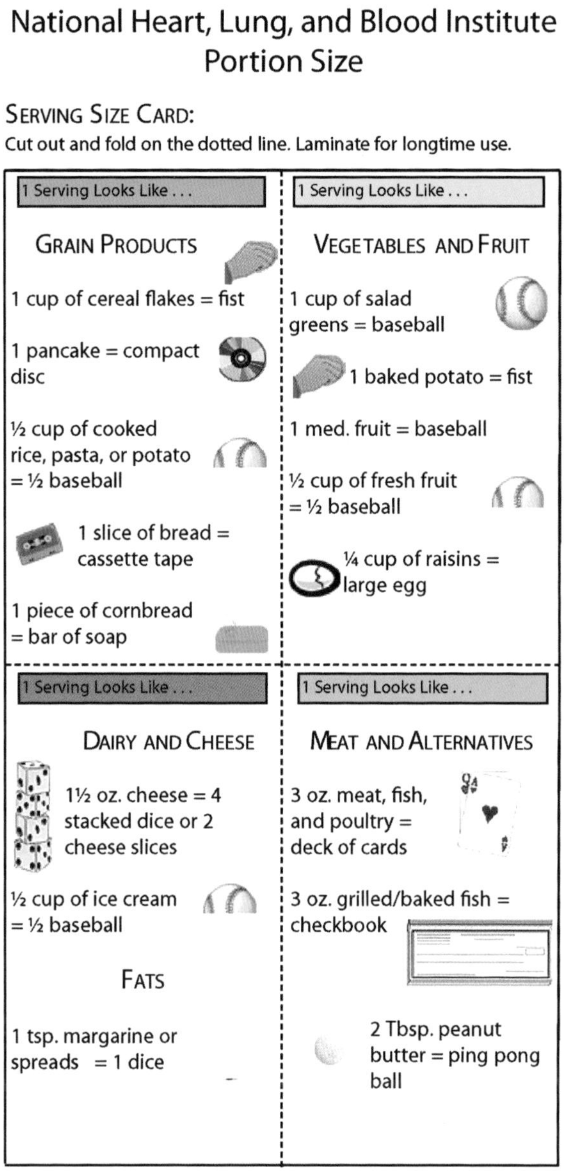

Fig. 9.11 Portion sizes
recommended by the
National Institute of Health.
Source: NHLBI [34]

National Heart, Lung, and Blood Institute Portion Size

SERVING SIZE CARD:

Cut out and fold on the dotted line. Laminate for longtime use.

1 Serving Looks Like . . .	1 Serving Looks Like . . .
GRAIN PRODUCTS	**VEGETABLES AND FRUIT**
1 cup of cereal flakes = fist	1 cup of salad greens = baseball
1 pancake = compact disc	1 baked potato = fist
½ cup of cooked rice, pasta, or potato = ½ baseball	1 med. fruit = baseball
1 slice of bread = cassette tape	½ cup of fresh fruit = ½ baseball
1 piece of cornbread = bar of soap	¼ cup of raisins = large egg

1 Serving Looks Like . . .	1 Serving Looks Like . . .
DAIRY AND CHEESE	**MEAT AND ALTERNATIVES**
1½ oz. cheese = 4 stacked dice or 2 cheese slices	3 oz. meat, fish, and poultry = deck of cards
½ cup of ice cream = ½ baseball	3 oz. grilled/baked fish = checkbook
FATS	
1 tsp. margarine or spreads = 1 dice	2 Tbsp. peanut butter = ping pong ball

Although snacking is a common source of overconsumption, it is not realistic or necessary to expect patients to eliminate all snacking, and I suggest preplanned specific snack sources to prevent overconsumption. Multiple MedDiet compatible snacks and suggestions are outlined in Chap. 16, and these should be available to consume if individuals are hungry between meals as alternatives to high calorie, unhealthy snack sources. It is better to consume a healthy, portion-controlled snack than to randomly grab the first, often high calorie, snack available when the urge

Table 9.3 Calories consumed away from home (Adapted from DGAC [1])

Changes in where we eat our food		
Food environment changes	Time frame	Percent change (%)
Percentage of meals and snacks eaten at fast food restaurants	1977–1995	200
Food at home expenditures as a share of disposable income	1970–2008	−42
Food away from home expenditures as a share of disposable income	1970–2008	26
Total food expenditures as a share of disposable income	1970–2008	−24

to snack becomes overwhelming. A key point for patients is that modern snack packaging has significantly increased in size and contents. Simply because a snack item is in a single bag, it does not mean that it is a single serving. Commercially prepared snacks can be split into two bags after purchase, with one consumed per snack time.

Location Meals: Homes Versus Fast Food

The second aspect of the current American food environment to address is the location of where people obtain their meals since this can have a significant effect on caloric intake. Food consumed away from home is more likely to be of higher caloric density and larger portion size than food consumed at home [1, 35]. Thus, it is not surprising that numerous studies have demonstrated that adults and children who regularly eat outside the home, particularly fast food, are at increased risk of weight gain and becoming overweight or obese [1, 25, 36–40]. Over the past several decades there has been a dramatic increase in the number of meals eaten away from home. Since 1970, the percent of annual food expenses incurred eating away from home increased from 26 to 42% [41], and the percentage of total calories consumed away from home increased from 18% in 1970 to 77% in 2010 [1] (Table 9.3 and Fig. 9.12). Encouraging patients to prepare and consume more meals at home can have a favorable impact on their weight status.

Energy Density

The third aspect of the current American food environment to address is its high energy density. Energy density is the amount of calories contained per unit of weight of a food. Dietary patterns that are higher in energy dense foods—such as foods comprised mostly of processed and refined carbohydrates and simple sugars—are associated with increased total energy intake and weight gain. High energy density

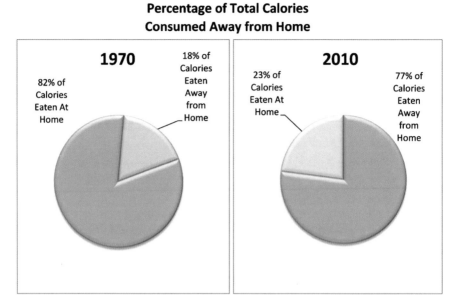

Fig. 9.12 Percentage of meals consumed away from home

foods lead to poor appetite control compared to the lower energy density foods found in a MedDiet, such as vegetables, fruits, and whole fiber products [1, 42–46]. It has also been demonstrated that decreasing the energy density of common foods such as pasta dishes and baked goods by adding pureed vegetables reduces total energy intake in ad libitum conditions [47]. This effective strategy will be shown in several recipes in Chap. 19.

A specific source of easily avoidable simple sugars is sweetened beverages. Unfortunately for our collective health, calories from beverages, both overall and as a percentage of total calories consumed, have been steadily increasing since the 1960s (Table 9.4). The percentage of total calories in the American diet that comes from beverages has increased from 12% of total energy intake in the 1970s to 21% today, or, on average, 220 more calories per day per person from beverages [38]. This problem is so pervasive that sugar or corn syrup sweetened beverages, such as sodas and sports drinks, are now the number one source of total caloric intake in individuals aged 14–30 years [15, 48]. A very simple, inexpensive way to slow down our obesity epidemic would be to substitute water or other noncaloric beverages for sugar-sweetened drinks.

Special Focus: Noncaloric Sweeteners

Noncaloric sweeteners are not considered in the calculation of a MedDiet-adherence score (AS). However, patients may ask about their potential effects on body weight

Table 9.4 Calories in beverages (adapted from DGAC[1])

Caloric value of common beverages		
Beverage	Standard serving size (fluid ounces)	Calories per serving size
Water	8	0
Water with teaspoon lime juice	8	1
Water with teaspoon lemon juice	8	1
Diet Cola	12	0
Cola	12	136
Sports drink	12	100
Juice drink	8	134
Apple juice	8	114
Orange juice	8	117
Tomato juice	6	31
Super-size Cola	24	270
Coffee	8	0
Tea	8	0

since there have been reports that use of noncaloric sweeteners may reduce the body's natural association of sweetness and energy and lead to overall excess caloric intake from other sources [49, 50]. By definition, if, in an otherwise identical controlled diet, caloric sweeteners are replaced with noncaloric sweeteners, the total energy contained in that diet will be reduced. There is no evidence this could cause anything but a relatively improved weight status. However, in free-living situations with ad libitum access to food, whether consumption of noncaloric sweeteners ultimately results in excess total caloric intake due to some mechanism stimulating overconsumption of other calorie sources during future meals is unclear. The most likely cause of any association between noncaloric sweeteners and overweight and obesity is simply that overweight people are more likely to seek out and consume noncaloric sweetened foods and beverages [1, 50–52].

Food Availability

The fourth component of the current American food environment to address is availability of healthy foods. Relative availability of food from generally unhealthy vendors such as convenience store or fast food establishments versus vendors selling fruits and vegetables affects health and weight. Living or working in close proximity to supermarkets or vendors that sell fruits and vegetables has been shown to reduce the incidence of overweight and obesity. Alternatively, close proximity to fast food and convenience stores, particularly when better alternatives are not nearby, has been shown to markedly increase rates of overweight and obesity [1, 53–56]. Studies have also shown that the availability of fruits and vegetables in the home increases the likelihood children will consume more of them and less unhealthy foods while increased availability of energy-dense foods in the home will increase their consumption [57, 58]. Creating a more healthy home food environment is discussed further in Chap. 16.

Daily Breakfast

A fifth and, perhaps not as immediately obvious, component of the food environment affecting overweight and obesity is the availability and consumption of a healthy breakfast most mornings. Numerous studies have shown that regularly skipping breakfast increases overweight and obesity while regular breakfast will decrease weight. This association is particularly strong for children and adolescents [1, 59–67].

Screen Time

The final part of the American food environment affecting overweight and obesity that should be addressed with patients is the time spent in front of television, video, or computer screens. There is a direct, positive association between screen time, especially television screen time, and overweight and obesity [1, 68–74]. There are many negative factors associated with increased screen time, such as exposure to ads for unhealthy foods, the common practice of concurrently consuming food while in front of a screen, and the physical inactivity when in front of a screen. Thus, individuals in front of television are often simultaneously consuming more and burning fewer calories while receiving marketing pitches for unhealthy food. This greatly increases the likelihood of a positive energy balance and weight gain.

A list of the areas in the food environment to address with patients when discussing ways to lose weight follows:

1. Portion size
2. Meals at home
3. Energy density
4. Healthy choices available
5. Regular breakfast
6. Screen time

Using a MedDiet for Weight Loss

This section of the chapter discusses using a MedDiet for weight loss and control, offers strategies for providers to use when working with patients for these purposes, and elaborates on the importance of regular physical activity both in weight loss and control and for general health.

A MedDiet is an effective tool for weight loss and control, but it is not a miracle weight loss diet. Such a diet never has, nor ever will, exist. It is important to maintain scientific rigor and reason when discussing dietary interventions for weight loss with patients. The statements made on the efficacy of the different diets discussed below are supported by the well-designed clinical studies to which they are referenced. Any data showing that a MedDiet helps with weight loss are, by definition, showing that it can be a useful way to achieve a negative energy balance. Patients must clearly understand that it is impossible for a MedDiet, or any diet, to be effective for weight loss if more calories are consumed than are burned. I like to have patients think of a MedDiet as offering a healthy, well-balanced variety of food choices that is both health promoting and effective for weight loss when consumed in a negative energy balance situation.

Comparison of Diets

When different macronutrients and macronutrient combinations are compared for effects on weight, they are all equivalent. Thus, although the foods one selects to consume can have very different effects on health, a calorie is a calorie for weight. Diet book authors have suggested that striking an "ideal" macronutrient balance—the percentage of fats, proteins, and carbohydrates in a diet—is important for effective weight loss. I commonly encounter patients who believe that some as-yet-untried combination of fats, carbohydrates, and proteins will make their excess pounds melt off. The reality is that no large well-designed clinical study has ever supported that macronutrient balance has an optimal ratio for weight loss. Indeed, whenever they have been compared over any significant period of time at isocaloric amounts, the macronutrient percentages in a diet are not associated with weight gain or loss [75–78]. In one analysis of the numerous published trials comparing high-fat, low-carbohydrate, moderate-fat, balanced-nutrient, low-fat, and very low-fat diets, each of these dietary strategies showed equivalent levels of weight loss at an equally negative energy balance. None were superior in any measured weight-effect criteria [79]. Additionally, in their review that evaluated 36 published studies on dietary macronutrient balance, the Dietary Guidelines for Americans Advisory Committee, 2010 concluded that, "There is strong and convincing evidence that when calorie intake is controlled, macronutrient proportion of the diet is not related to losing weight" [1]. Other systematic reviews of major studies looking specifically at low carbohydrate versus low-fat diets have also shown that in the published scientific literature there is no evidence of a difference in weight loss among different macronutrient balances over long-term follow-up [80–82]. The same conclusions that no diet is superior for weight loss at isocaloric amounts were published in other reviews that compared weight loss with the popular, branded diets: Atkins, Zone, Weight Watchers, Ornish, and Slimfast [83]. What all this means is that reaching a caloric deficit is the only mechanism for any diet to result in weight loss. The promotion of "newly discovered" variations on the theme of "ideal macronutrient balance" for weight loss is certain to continue, but the issue has been laid to rest from a scientific standpoint.

One question that I often address about using a MedDiet for weight loss is whether a diet that does not focus on restriction of calories from fat will make losing excess body fat more difficult. The macronutrient studies cited previously make it clear this is of no concern. Indeed, the robust use of plant-source fats such as olive oil in a MedDiet are, in addition to not adversely affecting weight control and body composition, an important source of the beneficial health effects of the dietary pattern [1, 84–86].

A MedDiet and a Mediterranean Enough Dietary Strategy

This section discusses how providers may improve patient results by recommending a MedDiet.

Obesity Trials

When reviewing obesity trials regarding a MedDiet, it is important to keep in mind that the single most important variable in a weight-loss diet's efficacy, other than ensuring a negative caloric balance has been achieved, is long-term adherence [1, 87]. Patients are more likely to be successful with caloric reduction when they like the food choices they are consuming; the variety of foods, less-restrictive rules, and highly palatable nature of a MedDiet enhance dietary adherence compared to other diets [82, 85, 88–91]. Several of the more important trials evaluating the use of a MedDiet for weight loss and control are outlined as follows:

In a study of more than 10,000 individuals using a nine category MedDiet-AS, those individuals with the lowest adherence scores (3 or less) had the highest average yearly weight gain while those with the highest adherence scores (6 or greater) had the lowest weight gain [92].

In a study of more than 27,000 participants followed for 3 years it was determined that, among those who were overweight at the beginning of the trial, those who had a high adherence to a MedDiet were 31% less likely to gain significant weight and become obese than those with a low MedDiet adherence. The authors concluded that a MedDiet might be useful to help combat obesity [93].

Four independent studies demonstrated that higher MedDiet adherence was associated with lower risk for obesity (range of 12–51% reduction) than a lower MedDiet adherence [94–97].

Six independent studies evaluating diet for weight loss showed a significantly greater reduction in weight in participants who were randomized to a Mediterranean diet versus those randomized to a control diet [85, 89, 98–101].

A large review looked at 21 major epidemiological studies that have assessed a MedDiet's effects on weight. The review's authors concluded that there might be a physiologic effect of the MedDiet to explain its observed benefits in the prevention of overweight and obesity. The authors urged more research to substantiate the promising association [102].

As there has recently been a reduction in adherence to a MedDiet in Mediterranean countries [103, 104] and adoption of a more Westernized diet, there has been a temporally associated rise in obesity levels. However, these levels are still significantly lower than obesity rates in Northern Europe and the United States [46].

A recent meta-analysis of 16 randomized controlled trials concluded that a MedDiet is useful for weight loss, especially when followed for 6 months or longer [105].

Office Steps for Clinicians

Clinicians are viewed as trusted sources of health information and can favorably influence healthy lifestyle habits [106]. There are several steps providers can take to help patients reduce overweight and obesity. When seeing patients in a clinic setting, they should be weighed at every visit with body weight and BMI being considered vital signs that are just as important to check at routine visits as is blood pressure. If overweight or obesity is diagnosed, these should be addressed as modifiable diseases that are detrimental to health. Then, patients who are overweight or obese should be instructed to start a daily log for self-monitoring food intake, physical activity, and body weight. Regular recording in a daily log has been shown to change behaviors and result in better long-term outcomes [1]. Additionally, at follow-up visits, providers should review any self-monitoring logs a patient is keeping and record results for comparison. Frequent office follow-up has also been shown to increase compliance with physician-recommended diet and lifestyle changes [1, 107–111]. In summary, the office steps to take to improve the efficacy of a MedDiet for weight management are:

1. Try to be a role model for patients.
2. Weigh and calculate BMI at each office visit.
3. Discuss health risks of overweight and obesity.
4. Assist with log for recording meals, activity, and weight.
5. Schedule frequent office follow-up to improve compliance.

Physicians have actually been spending less time counseling patients on weight control than in past decades [112]. One telling ambulatory care survey revealed that 63% of patients with a BMI of greater than 30, the level for obesity, had received no dietary, exercise, or weight-loss counseling from their physicians [113]. There are challenges physicians encounter when attempting to assist patients with weight loss. In one study, the majority of physicians surveyed reported a lack of time to counsel patients on overweight and obesity as an impediment to success.

Additionally, they noted a lack of simple, effective, and trustworthy recommendations that they could use in the office setting for assistance with this task [114]. Another barrier is that as societies have become more overweight, people's perception about what a healthy body weight looks like has changed. Fewer people today actually think of themselves as overweight than they would have in past decades [115] even though the burdens of overweight and obesity have dramatically increased.

Starting a Program

The critical concept for patients to understand regarding dieting for weight control is energy balance. For weight maintenance, they must keep energy intake and expenditure at equal amounts for years on end. For weight loss, a negative energy balance from vigilant regulation of the food and beverages they consume and maintaining daily activity levels is necessary. Frequent monitoring of weight will give patients feedback on what their energy balance is.

I have found that giving patients target numbers can be useful when working together on a weight loss program. When initiating caloric restriction for weight loss, I recommended starting women at a level of 1,000–1,200 cal/day and men at 1,200–1,600 cal/day. An alternative strategy is to have patients log the calories from their current diet over a period of 1 week and then reduce their daily average by 500–1,000 cal/day. These recommended calorie levels should be adjusted at follow-up visits as weight loss, compliance issues, exercise levels, and hunger tolerance require. Total calories consumed should always come from a well-balanced meal plan and should never go below 800 cal/day except at facilities with medical experts experienced in managing a very-low-calorie diet closely supervising the patients.

Patients often have unrealistic expectations for how rapidly they will lose weight when I see them in the clinic. Although it is important to not dampen their enthusiasm, it is equally important to be an honest broker of the truth. By the time patients are working with me for weight loss, they have often unsuccessfully tried several other programs and read numerous popular diet books that have overpromised results. I tell patients that a reasonable expectation when using a MedDiet for weight loss at the caloric levels noted previously is a rate of loss of 1–2 lb/week over the first 4–12 weeks. After that, the rate will likely slow to 0.5–1 lb/week. These numbers are based on my experience with hundreds of patients and on National Institutes of Health (NIH) data that show a caloric deficit of 500 cal/day results in approximately 1 lb/week of nonwater weight loss [116]. Once an individual has achieved a loss of 10% of body weight and has been able to maintain this new weight for at least 6 months, further caloric reduction and increases in activity may be implemented for additional weight loss. Many patients would love to see fat melt off more quickly, but that simply is not realistic and they must be advised so. Using a multiyear calendar diagram is helpful in communicating the fact that slow yet continuous rates of weight loss add up to very to substantial, life-changing levels. With a modest 1 lb of loss per month for 12 months, over the course of 4 years

Conceptual Calendar Showing Cumulative Weight Loss over Time

Start Weight = 242 lbs   Rate of weight loss: 1 lb per month

Year 2007			
Jan	Feb	Mar	Apr
242	241	240	239
May	Jun	Jul	Aug
238	237	236	235
Sep	Oct	Nov	Dec
234	233	232	231

Year 2009			
Jan	Feb	Mar	Apr
218	217	216	215
May	Jun	Jul	Aug
214	213	212	211
Sep	Oct	Nov	Dec
210	209	208	207

Year 2008			
Jan	Feb	Mar	Apr
230	229	228	227
May	Jun	Jul	Aug
226	225	224	223
Sep	Oct	Nov	Dec
222	221	220	219

Year 2010			
Jan	Feb	Mar	Apr
206	205	204	203
May	Jun	Jul	Aug
202	201	200	199
Sep	Oct	Nov	Dec
198	197	196	195*

* Realistic Expectation for new
life-long weight

Fig. 9.13 Calendar diagram of cumulative weight loss over time

patients would achieve a nearly 50-lb weight loss (Fig. 9.13). Chapters 16, 17, and 19 contain meal planning, food ideas, and recipes with palatable and convenient MedDiet foods for weight loss and control.

For Weight Loss Plan

1. Initiate at 1,000–1,200 cal/day in women and 1,200–1,600 cal/day in men.
2. May initiate at 500–1,000 cal/day below current daily average.
3. Maintain daily physical activity.
4. Set realistic expectations for rate of weight loss, think long-term to life-long.
5. Keep log of daily food, activity, and weight.
6. Adjust intake and activity as indicated.

Physical Activity

Physical activity is necessary for both weight control and overall health. For patients to have success at long-term weight control, they should be helped to find an activity regimen they can realistically sustain in their daily lives. In addition to reducing overweight and obesity, higher levels of physical activity reduce the risk for heart attacks, strokes, type 2 diabetes (T2D), hypertension, and metabolic syndrome [117–121]. Alternatively, a sedentary lifestyle has been shown to increase premature

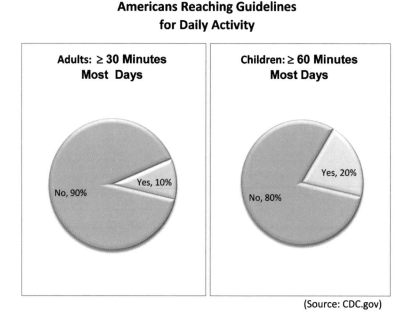

Fig. 9.14 Pie charts showing percentage of Americans meeting the daily activity guidelines. *Source*: CDC [6]

death, cardiovascular diseases, hypertension T2D, osteoporosis, cancer, and depression [122–125]. If patients are not regularly active then they are failing at a key component of disease prevention and longevity promotion.

The vast majority of Americans do not come close to enough daily activity to benefit from its health promoting and weight loss effects. Current guidelines recommend physical activity of moderate to vigorous level for 60 min in adolescents and 30 min in adults at least 5 days/week [6] (Fig. 9.14). Recent surveys have shown that only 5% of adults meet these guidelines and that more than 32% of females and 18% of males are never physically active for 30 min even once per week [126–128].

The data for physical activity in children are equally discouraging. Only 8% of American children age 12–19 meet the guidelines for 60 min or more of physical activity at least 5 days/week [128]. This is not because of lack of free time since more than 50% of American youth report greater than 3 h/day of watching television [129]. The priorities are just not set properly. There is a direct correlation between more screen time and reduced physical activity [130, 131]. For parents, one way to intervene is to require physical activity prior to any day's screen time.

Screen time also increases mortality risk in adults. Television viewing has been shown in a large trial to have a direct effect on mortality with an 11% increase in mortality rate for each hour spent watching television [132]. This is almost certainly because television viewing is a marker for inactivity and not due to some disease inducing effect of television per se.

As these numbers for physical activity levels demonstrate, we are doing a poor job of reaching recommended levels of physical activity in both children and adults. Health care providers can have some impact on this by making a physical activity survey part of routine visits: ask about physical activity levels at every patient encounter, request patients keep a physical activity log and bring it with them to appointments, and offer suggestions for incorporating physical activity into daily routines. This is just as important to health as asking about chronic conditions, medications, and screening test status. Since there is no pill or other alternative to physical activity, we simply must get our patients moving more. Some practical measures to increase activity are presented in the discussion that follows.

Activities Available

For a sedentary person to become active, he or she must find some activity or activities that can and will realistically be incorporated into daily life. Significant interpersonal variability exists in interests, physical limitations, and in daily life constraints so presenting a list of numerous practical options can be helpful. Patients may find it is easier than anticipated to reach a minimum of 30 min of activity per day if told that it may be broken into two 15 or three 10-min daily segments, as the time spent in activity does not have to be one continuous effort to be effective.

When counseling most patients for beginning an activity regimen, I start with showing them the list in Table 9.5 of simple and easy to incorporate forms of daily activity. I use terms "incorporating daily physical activity" rather than "getting you on a good exercise regimen" with my more sedentary patients. As providers, we need to remember that we are not training our patients for the Olympics; our goal is simply to get them moving more every day. I have found that overly ambitious regimens, either from the patient or provider, are more likely to be completely dropped in a few months than more modest plans. I tell patients that although the activities on the list are simple and not overly strenuous, they must be done every day. Once they have achieved compliance for at least several weeks at 30 min/day, they can then start adding more time if desired.

A list of activities from which to mix and match follows, but first a brief outline of the nearly ideal activity, walking, is presented. Walking is one of the easiest to start and most convenient and highly portable of all forms of physical activity. Effort and pace are individual driven and can be increased as fitness allows. A simple tactic I advise that may be used nearly anywhere is to walk 15 min out the door, turnaround, and return. When working from home, one can break every hour or two and take a quick 5-min walk around the block, which often results in enhanced concentration and performance on returning to work. This can also be done from home, office, in airports, in large buildings, and while traveling.

Table 9.5 Appropriate calories burned per 30 min in common activities

Activity	Calories burned[a]
Walking	
Leisurely: 2 mph	85
Briskly: 4 mph	170
Gardening	135
Raking leaves	145
Dancing	190
Social	150
Bicycling	
Leisurely: 10 mph	205
Moderately: 15 mph	250
Aggressively: 20 mph	350
Swimming laps	
Medium effort	240
Hard effort	325
Jogging	
Slowly: 5 mph	275
Medium: 7.5 mph	350
Very fast: 10 mph	510
Golf, carrying clubs	200
Wash and wax car	225
Shovel snow	300
Stair walking	300
Basketball game (vigorous full court)	400

Source: NHLBI, 2010 [34]

The greater the intensity for any of these activities, the more calories that will be burned

[a]For 150 lb. person; a lighter person burns fewer calories, a heavier person more

Another simple way to walk more is to park farther away from work or get off public transport farther from work so there is no option but to increase activity levels at the start and end of the day. Walking a few flights of stairs at work once or twice daily, perhaps after a meeting or at the start of a break or beginning of the workday are also very accessible options. I suggest people who are working from home and have stairs in their house take a break about every hour to walk up and down the stairs twice. Intermittently standing while working has been shown to significantly increase caloric expenditure [133]. Some people are able to move their work to the top of a cabinet or dresser or designated stand up desk. Another popular choice to increase activity is to join or form a daily lunch walk group at work. The two tables that follow show the number of calories burned per hour for common activities (Table 9.5) and a list of activities that patients can mix and match to obtain their 30 min of activity daily (Table 9.6).

Table 9.6 Suggestions to increase daily activity

Walking
  Walk outdoors 15 min, return
  Walk around block each morning before breakfast
  Park at least 0.5 miles from office
  Get off public transit 1 stop earlier
  Walk at office lunch, alone or in group
  Take stairs at start, middle, breaks, and/or end of day at home or office
  Walk around block before and after eating out or at home
  Take walk during one–one meetings
  Stand/walk while on telephone
Stationary exercise
  Exercise bike, treadmill, or elliptical machine at home
  Dumbbells at home or office, use every 2 h throughout the day
  Occasionally work standing up
Outdoor and about
  Bike to work
  Park farther away at work, at stores
  Walk or bike for trips under 1 mile
  Bike ride
  Jog or run
  Walk while golfing
  Basketball
  Racquetball
  Lift weights
  Dance
  Aerobics, exercise classes
  Yoga class
At home
  Walk stairs frequently
  Walk around block before/after dinner
  Garden, yard work
  Wash and wax car
  Housework
  Stationary bike or treadmill when watching television
  Stand up/walk while on phone
  Shovel snow

Insurance Coverage for Screening and Counseling for Obesity

A New and Exciting Development for Providers Combating the Obesity Epidemic: Removing the Obstacle of Lack of Reimbursement

On November 29, 2011, the Centers for Medicare and Medicaid Services (CMS) announced that Medicare would add coverage for preventive services to reduce obesity [134]. As part of this announcement, CMS Administrator Donald M. Berwick, MD stated, "Obesity is a challenge faced by Americans of all ages, and prevention is crucial for the management and elimination of obesity in our country. It is important for Medicare patients to enjoy access to appropriate preventive services" [134].

Although this insurance coverage only applies to Medicare at the time of writing this book, private insurers nearly always follow Medicare's lead on adding screening benefits, and the barrier of lack of reimbursement as a disincentive to providers spending time counseling their patients on healthy dieting for weight loss and control may become a problem of the past.

As part of their decision summary [135], CMS cited US Preventive Services Task Force (USPSTF) findings that intensive behavioral therapy for obesity, defined as a BMI of 30 kg/m², is reasonable and necessary for the prevention or early detection of illness or disability. The CMS guidelines define intensive behavioral therapy for obesity as consisting of the following [135]:

1. Screening for obesity in adults using measurement of BMI calculated by dividing weight in kilograms by the square of height in meters (expressed in kg/m²).
2. Dietary (nutritional) assessment.
3. Intensive behavioral counseling and behavioral therapy to promote sustained weight loss through high intensity interventions on diet and exercise.

The CMS guidelines further state that the intensive behavioral intervention for obesity should be consistent with the "5-A" framework—Assess, Advise, Agree, Assist, Arrange—highlighted by the USPSTF [135]:

1. Assess: Ask about/assess behavioral health risk(s) and factors affecting choice of behavior change goals/methods.
2. Advise: Give clear, specific, and personalized behavior change advice, including information about personal health harms and benefits.
3. Agree: Collaboratively select appropriate treatment goals and methods based on the patient's interest in and willingness to change behavior.
4. Assist: Using behavior change techniques (self-help and/or counseling), aid the patient in achieving agreed-upon goals by acquiring the skills, confidence, and social/environmental supports for behavior change, supplemented with adjunctive medical treatments when appropriate.
5. Arrange: Schedule follow-up contacts (in person or by telephone) to provide ongoing assistance/support and to adjust the treatment plan as needed, including referral to more intensive or specialized treatment.

The CMS decision memo also states that for Medicare beneficiaries with obesity, who are competent and alert at the time that counseling is provided and whose counseling is furnished by a qualified primary care physician or other primary care practitioner and in a primary care setting, CMS covers [135]:

- One face-to-face visit every week for the first month.
- One face-to-face visit every other week for months 2–6.
- One face-to-face visit every month for months 7–12, if the beneficiary meets the 3-kg weight loss requirement as discussed as follows.

> **Medicare's Coverage of Screening and Counseling for Obesity:**
> **Primary Care Provider's Patient Encounter Check List**

☑ = done

☐ Determined patient's BMI is >= 30 kg/m2

☐ Performed dietary (nutritional) assessment

☐ Performed intensive behavioral counseling and behavioral therapy to promote sustained weight loss through high-intensity interventions on diet and exercise.

☐ Ensured when performing intensive behavioral intervention for obesity it was consistent with the "5-A framework" as listed below:

⊘ = done

◯ Assessed: Asked about/assessed behavioral health risk(s) and factors affecting choice of behavior change goals/methods.

◯ Advised: Gave clear, specific, and personalized behavior change advice, including information about personal health harms and benefits.

◯ Agreed: Collaboratively selected appropriate treatment goals and methods based on the patient's interest in and willingness to change behavior.

◯ Assisted: Used behavior change techniques (self-help and/or counseling) to aid the patient in achieving agreed-upon goals by acquiring the skills, confidence, and social/environmental supports for behavior change, supplemented with adjunctive medical treatments when appropriate.

◯ Arranged: Scheduled follow-up contacts (in person or by telephone) to provide ongoing assistance/support and to adjust the treatment plan as needed, including referral to more intensive or specialized treatment.

☐ Counseling was provided by primary care practitioner in a primary care setting.

☐ Counseling was provided within or less frequently than schedule of:

■ One face-to-face visit every week for the first month
■ One face-to-face visit every other week for months 2-6
■ One face-to-face visit every month for months 7-12, if the beneficiary has achieved a 3 kg weight loss at the month 6 visit

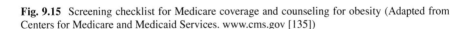

Fig. 9.15 Screening checklist for Medicare coverage and counseling for obesity (Adapted from Centers for Medicare and Medicaid Services. www.cms.gov [135])

At the 6-month visit, a reassessment of obesity and a determination of the amount of weight loss must be performed. To be eligible for additional face-to-face visits occurring once a month for an additionally 6 months, beneficiaries must have achieved a reduction in weight of at least 3 kg over the course of the first 6 months of intensive therapy. This determination must be documented in the physician office records for applicable beneficiaries consistent with usual practice. For beneficiaries who do not achieve a weight loss of at least 3 kg during the first

6 months of intensive therapy, a reassessment of their readiness to change and BMI is appropriate after an additional 6-month period [135] (Fig. 9.15).

Health care providers may find that they can use the information contained throughout this book to assist them in providing their patients with the "intensive behavioral therapy for obesity" that is now a covered Medicare benefit and will likely soon be a covered benefit of private insurers. The public health benefits of this forward thinking move by CMS to cover preventive services may be significant.

Conclusion

I have found it effective when counseling patients on controlling caloric intake and maintaining daily activity to inform them that the effort required may be challenging at first, but the longer they sustain the effort, the more it will feel like a natural and integral part of their day (Table 9.7). Initially, they may need to consciously start the day with:

"Today, I do not consume excess calories" and "Today, I will be more active."

But these can quickly morph into:

"I am someone who does not consume excess calories" and "I always get extra activity in my day."

Ultimately, they become part of who a person is. Controlling calories is not a destination; it is a lifelong journey.

Table 9.7 Actions to address and control weight

Physician's office assessment
Act as a role model
Weigh and calculate BMI each visit
Address health risk of overweight and obesity
Advise keeping a log for food, activity, and weight
Have patients schedule frequent follow-ups
Control the food environment
Reduce portion sizes
Prepare and eat more meals at home
Choose foods of lower energy density
Keep healthy options available
Eat breakfast daily
Reduce screen time
Execute weight loss plan
Initiate at 1,000–1,200 cal/day in women; 1,200–1,600 cal/day for men
May also initiate at 500–1,000 cal/day below current daily average
Maintain daily physical activity
Have realistic expectations for rate of loss; think long-term to lifelong
Keep log of daily food, activity, and weight
Adjust intake and activity as indicated

References

1. Dietary Guidelines for Americans Committee; U.S. Department of Agriculture. Center for Nutrition Policy and Promotion. Dietary guidelines for Americans, 2010. http://www.cnpp. usda.gov/dietaryguidelines.htm. Accessed 1 Jan 2011.
2. Daniels SR, Jacobson MS, McCrindle BW, Eckel RH, Sanner BM. American Heart Association Childhood Obesity Research Summit: executive summary. Circulation. 2009;119(15):2114–23.
3. Gilliland FD, Berhane K, Islam T, McConnell R, Gauderman WJ, Gilliland SS, Avol E, Peters JM. Obesity and the risk of newly diagnosed asthma in school-age children. Am J Epidemiol. 2003;158(5):406–15.
4. Pi-Sunyer X. The medical risks of obesity. Postgrad Med. 2009;121(6):21–33.
5. Rofey DL, Kolko RP, Iosif AM, Silk JS, Bost JE, Feng W, et al. A longitudinal study of childhood depression and anxiety in relation to weight gain. Child Psychiatry Hum Dev. 2009;40(4):517–26.
6. Centers for Disease Control. National Center for Health Statistics (NCHS). http://www.cdc. gov/nchs/. Accessed 27 May 2011.
7. Flegal KM, Carroll MD, Ogden CL, Curtin LR. Prevalence and trends in obesity among US adults, 1999-2008. JAMA. 2010;303(3):235–41.
8. Ogden CL, Carroll MD, Curtin LR, Lamb MM, Flegal KM. Prevalence of high body mass index in US children and adolescents, 2007-2008. JAMA. 2010;303(3):242–9.
9. Ogden CL, Carroll MD, Flegal KM. High body mass index for age among US children and adolescents, 2003-2006. JAMA. 2008;299(20):2401–5.
10. US Department of Health and Human Services. The Surgeon General's call to action to prevent overweight and obesity: overweight in children and adolescents. Washington, DC: US Department of Health and Human Services; 2007.
11. Singh AS, Mulder C, Twisk JW, van Mechelen W, Chinapaw MJ. Tracking of childhood overweight into adulthood: a systematic review of the literature. Obes Rev. 2008;9(5): 474–88.
12. Mission: Readiness—Military Leaders for Kids. Too fat to fight: retired military leaders want junk food out of America's schools. New York: Mission Readiness; 2010.
13. Must A, Jacques PF, Dallal GE, Bajema CJ, Dietz WH. Long-term morbidity and mortality of overweight adolescents. A follow-up of the Harvard Growth Study of 1922 to 1935. N Engl J Med. 1992;327(19):1350–5.
14. Latner JD, Stunkard AJ, Wilson GT. Stigmatized students: age, sex, and ethnicity effects in the stigmatization of obesity. Obes Res. 2005;13(7):1226–31.
15. Wang Y, Beydoun MA, Liang L, Caballero B, Kumanyika SK. Will all Americans become overweight or obese? Estimating the progression and cost of the US obesity epidemic. Obesity (Silver Spring). 2008;16(10):2323–30.
16. Finkelstein EA, Trogdon JG, Cohen JW, Dietz W. Annual medical spending attributable to obesity: payer-and service-specific estimates. Health Aff (Millwood). 2009;28(5):w822–31.
17. Nielsen SJ, Popkin BM. Patterns and trends in food portion sizes, 1977-1998. JAMA. 2003;289(4):450–3.
18. Mellen PB, Gao SK, Vitolins MZ, Goff Jr DC. Deteriorating dietary habits among adults with hypertension: DASH dietary accordance, NHANES 1988-1994 and 1999-2004. Arch Intern Med. 2008;168(3):308–14.
19. Ello-Martin JA, Ledikwe JH, Rolls BJ. The influence of food portion size and energy density on energy intake: implications for weight management. Am J Clin Nutr. 2005; 82(1 Suppl):236S–41.
20. Fisher JO, Kral TV. Super-size me: portion size effects on young children's eating. Physiol Behav. 2008;94(1):39–47.
21. Malik VS, Schulze MB, Hu FB. Intake of sugar-sweetened beverages and weight gain: a systematic review. Am J Clin Nutr. 2006;84(2):274–88.

22. Sichieri R, Paula Trotte A, de Souza RA, Veiga GV. School randomised trial on prevention of excessive weight gain by discouraging students from drinking sodas. Public Health Nutr. 2009;12(2):197–202.
23. Bowman SA, Vinyard BT. Fast food consumption of U.S. adults: impact on energy and nutrient intakes and overweight status. J Am Coll Nutr. 2004;23(2):163–8.
24. Kant AK, Graubard BI. Eating out in America, 1987-2000: trends and nutritional correlates. Prev Med. 2004;38(2):243–9.
25. Rosenheck R. Fast food consumption and increased caloric intake: a systematic review of a trajectory towards weight gain and obesity risk. Obes Rev. 2008;9(6):535–47.
26. Gilhooly CH, Das SK, Golden JK, McCrory MA, Dallal GE, Saltzman E, Kramer FM, Roberts SB. Food cravings and energy regulation: the characteristics of craved foods and their relationship with eating behaviors and weight change during 6 months of dietary energy restriction. Int J Obes (Lond). 2007;31(12):1849–58.
27. Hannum SM, Carson LA, Evans EM, Petr EL, Wharton CM, Bui L, Erdman Jr JW. Use of packaged entrees as part of a weight-loss diet in overweight men: an 8-week randomized clinical trial. Diabetes Obes Metab. 2006;8(2):146–55.
28. Pearcey SM, de Castro JM. Food intake and meal patterns of weight-stable and weight-gaining persons. Am J Clin Nutr. 2002;76(1):107–12.
29. Rolls BJ, Morris EL, Roe LS. Portion size of food affects energy intake in normal-weight and overweight men and women. Am J Clin Nutr. 2002;76(6):1207–13.
30. Rolls BJ, Roe LS, Kral TV, Meengs JS, Wall DE. Increasing the portion size of a packaged snack increases energy intake in men and women. Appetite. 2004;42(1):63–9.
31. Diliberti N, Bordi PL, Conklin MT, Roe LS, Rolls BJ. Increased portion size leads to increased energy intake in a restaurant meal. Obes Res. 2004;12(3):562–8.
32. Wansink B, Park SB. At the movies: how external cues and perceived taste impact consumption volume. J Database Marketing. 1996;60:1–14.
33. Wansink B, Cheney MM. Super bowls: serving bowl size and food consumption. JAMA. 2005;293(14):1727–8.
34. National Heart Lung and Blood Institute (NHLBI) portion size. http://hin.nhlbi.nih.gov/portion/servingcard7.pdf. Accessed May 27, 2011.
35. Guthrie JF, Lin BH, Frazao E. Role of food prepared away from home in the American diet, 1977-78 versus 1994-96: changes and consequences. J Nutr Educ Behav. 2002;34(3):140–50.
36. Taveras EM, Berkey CS, Rifas-Shiman SL, Ludwig DS, Rockett HR, Field AE, et al. Association of consumption of fried food away from home with body mass index and diet quality in older children and adolescents. Pediatrics. 2005;116(4):e518–24.
37. Thompson OM, Ballew C, Resnicow K, Must A, Bandini LG, Cyr H, Dietz WH. Food purchased away from home as a predictor of change in BMI z-score among girls. Int J Obes Relat Metab Disord. 2004;28(2):282–9.
38. Duffey KJ, Gordon-Larsen P, Jacobs Jr DR, Williams OD, Popkin BM. Differential associations of fast food and restaurant food consumption with 3-y change in body mass index: the Coronary Artery Risk Development in Young Adults Study. Am J Clin Nutr. 2007;85(1):201–8.
39. Li F, Harmer P, Cardinal BJ, Bosworth M, Johnson-Shelton D, Moore JM, et al. Built environment and 1-year change in weight and waist circumference in middle-aged and older adults: Portland Neighborhood Environment and Health Study. Am J Epidemiol. 2009;169(4):401–8.
40. Pereira MA, Kartashov AI, Ebbeling CB, Van Horn L, Slattery ML, Jacobs DR, Jr., Ludwig DS. Fast-food habits, weight gain, and insulin resistance (the CARDIA study): 15-year prospective analysis. Lancet. 2005;365(9453):36-42. Erratum in: Lancet. 2005;365(9464):1030.
41. National Center for Health Statistics (US). Health, United States, 2008: with special feature on the health of young adults. Hyattsville, MD: National Center for Health Statistics (US); 2009.

42. Erlanson-Albertsson C. How palatable food disrupts appetite regulation. Basic Clin Pharmacol Toxicol. 2005;97(2):61–73.
43. Rolls BJ. The relationship between dietary energy density and energy intake. Physiol Behav. 2009;97(5):609–15.
44. Ledikwe JH, Rolls BJ, Smiciklas-Wright H, Mitchell DC, Ard JD, Champagne C, Karanja N, Lin PH, Stevens VJ, Appel LJ. Reductions in dietary energy density are associated with weight loss in overweight and obese participants in the PREMIER trial. Am J Clin Nutr. 2007;85(5):1212–21.
45. Savage JS, Marini M, Birch LL. Dietary energy density predicts women's weight change over 6 y. Am J Clin Nutr. 2008;88(3):677–84.
46. Schröder H. Protective mechanisms of the Mediterranean diet in obesity and type 2 diabetes. J Nutr Biochem. 2007;18(3):149–60.
47. Blatt AD, Roe LS, Rolls BJ. Hidden vegetables: an effective strategy to reduce energy intake and increase vegetable intake in adults. Am J Clin Nutr. 2011;93(4):756–63.
48. National Cancer Institute. Usual dietary intakes: food intakes, US population, 2004-2010. http://riskfactor.cancer.gov/diet/usualintakes/pop/.
49. Swithers SE, Baker CR, Davidson TL. General and persistent effects of high-intensity sweeteners on body weight gain and caloric compensation in rats. Behav Neurosci. 2009;123(4):772–80.
50. Fowler SP, Williams K, Resendez RG, Hunt KJ, Hazuda HP, Stern MP. Fueling the obesity epidemic? Artificially sweetened beverage use and long-term weight gain. Obesity (Silver Spring). 2008;16(8):1894–900.
51. American Diabetes Association. http://www.diabetes.org/news-research/research/?loc= DropDownNR-research. Accessed Nov 23, 2011.
52. Flood JE, Roe LS, Rolls BJ. The effect of increased beverage portion size on energy intake at a meal. J Am Diet Assoc. 2006;106(12):1984–90; discussion 1990–1.
53. Ford PB, Dzewaltowski DA. Disparities in obesity prevalence due to variation in the retail food environment: three testable hypotheses. Nutr Rev. 2008;66(4):216–28.
54. Giskes K, Kamphuis CB, van Lenthe FJ, Kremers S, Droomers M, Brug J. A systematic review of associations between environmental factors, energy and fat intakes among adults: is there evidence for environments that encourage obesogenic dietary intakes? Public Health Nutr. 2007;10(10):1005–17.
55. Holsten JE. Obesity and the community food environment: a systematic review. Public Health Nutr. 2009;12(3):397–405.
56. van der Horst K, Oenema A, Ferreira I, Wendel-Vos W, Giskes K, van Lenthe F, Brug J. A systematic review of environmental correlates of obesity-related dietary behaviors in youth. Health Educ Res. 2007;22(2):203–26.
57. Resnicow K, Davis-Hearn M, Smith M, Baranowski T, Lin LS, Baranowski J, Doyle C, Wang DT. Social-cognitive predictors of fruit and vegetable intake in children. Health Psychol. 1997;16(3):272–6.
58. Domel SB, Baranowski T, Davis HC, Thompson WO, Leonard SB, Baranowski J. A measure of stages of change in fruit and vegetable consumption among fourth- and fifth-grade school children: reliability and validity. J Am Coll Nutr. 1996;15(1):56–64.
59. Ask AS, Hernes S, Aarek I, Johannessen G, Haugen M. Changes in dietary pattern in 15 year old adolescents following a 4 month dietary intervention with school breakfast—a pilot study. Nutr J. 2006;5:33.
60. Albertson AM, Franko DL, Thompson D, Eldridge AL, Holschuh N, Affenito SG, et al. Longitudinal patterns of breakfast eating in black and white adolescent girls. Obesity (Silver Spring). 2007;15(9):2282–92.
61. Barton BA, Eldridge AL, Thompson D, Affenito SG, Striegel-Moore RH, Franko DL, Albertson AM, Crockett SJ. The relationship of breakfast and cereal consumption to nutrient intake and body mass index: the National Heart, Lung, and Blood Institute Growth and Health Study. J Am Diet Assoc. 2005;105(9):1383–9.

62. Crossman A, Anne Sullivan D, Benin M. The family environment and American adolescents' risk of obesity as young adults. Soc Sci Med. 2006;63(9):2255–67.
63. Elgar FJ, Roberts C, Moore L, Tudor-Smith C. Sedentary behaviour, physical activity and weight problems in adolescents in Wales. Public Health. 2005;119(6):518–24.
64. Haines J, Neumark-Sztainer D, Wall M, Story M. Personal, behavioral, and environmental risk and protective factors for adolescent overweight. Obesity (Silver Spring). 2007;15(11): 2748–60.
65. Merten MJ, Williams AL, Shriver LH. Breakfast consumption in adolescence and young adulthood: parental presence, community context, and obesity. J Am Diet Assoc. 2009;109(8):1384–91.
66. Niemeier HM, Raynor HA, Lloyd-Richardson EE, Rogers ML, Wing RR. Fast food consumption and breakfast skipping: predictors of weight gain from adolescence to adulthood in a nationally representative sample. J Adolesc Health. 2006;39(6):842–9.
67. Timlin MT, Pereira MA, Story M, Neumark-Sztainer D. Breakfast eating and weight change in a 5-year prospective analysis of adolescents: Project EAT (Eating Among Teens). Pediatrics. 2008;121(3):e638–45.
68. Marshall SJ, Biddle SJ, Gorely T, Cameron N, Murdey I. Relationships between media use, body fatness and physical activity in children and youth: a meta-analysis. Int J Obes Relat Metab Disord. 2004;28(10):1238–46.
69. Hancox RJ, Milne BJ, Poulton R. Association between child and adolescent television viewing and adult health: a longitudinal birth cohort study. Lancet. 2004;364(9430):257–62.
70. Hu FB, Li TY, Colditz GA, Willett WC, Manson JE. Television watching and other sedentary behaviors in relation to risk of obesity and type 2 diabetes mellitus in women. JAMA. 2003;289(14):1785–91.
71. Oken E, Taveras EM, Popoola FA, Rich-Edwards JW, Gillman MW. Television, walking, and diet: associations with postpartum weight retention. Am J Prev Med. 2007;32(4):305–11.
72. Parsons TJ, Manor O, Power C. Television viewing and obesity: a prospective study in the 1958 British birth cohort. Eur J Clin Nutr. 2008;62(12):1355–63.
73. Raynor DA, Phelan S, Hill JO, Wing RR. Television viewing and long-term weight maintenance: results from the National Weight Control Registry. Obesity (Silver Spring). 2006;14(10):1816–24.
74. Viner RM, Cole TJ. Television viewing in early childhood predicts adult body mass index. J Pediatr. 2005;147(4):429–35.
75. Willett WC. Dietary fat plays a major role in obesity: no. Obes Rev. 2002;3(2):59–68.
76. Willett WC, Leibel RL. Dietary fat is not a major determinant of body fat. Am J Med. 2002;113(Suppl 9B):47S–59.
77. Brehm BJ, D'Alessio DA. Weight loss and metabolic benefits with diets of varying fat and carbohydrate content: separating the wheat from the chaff. Nat Clin Pract Endocrinol Metab. 2008;4(3):140–6.
78. van Dam RM, Seidell JC. Carbohydrate intake and obesity. Eur J Clin Nutr. 2007;61 Suppl 1:S75–99.
79. Freedman MR, King J, Kennedy E. Popular diets: a scientific review. Obes Res. 2001;9 Suppl 1:1S–40.
80. Pirozzo S, Summerbell C, Cameron C, Glasziou P. Advice on low-fat diets for obesity. Cochrane Database Syst Rev. 2002;(2):CD003640. Review. Update in: Cochrane Database Syst Rev. 2008;(3):CD003640.
81. Bravata DM, Sanders L, Huang J, Krumholz HM, Olkin I, Gardner CD, Bravata DM. Efficacy and safety of low-carbohydrate diets: a systematic review. JAMA. 2003;289(14):1837–50.
82. Nordmann AJ, Nordmann A, Briel M, Keller U, Yancy Jr WS, Brehm BJ, Bucher HC. Effects of low-carbohydrate vs low-fat diets on weight loss and cardiovascular risk factors: a meta-analysis of randomized controlled trials. Arch Intern Med. 2006;166(3):285–93.
83. Truby H, Baic S, deLooy A, Fox KR, Livingstone MB, Logan CM, et al. Randomised controlled trial of four commercial weight loss programmes in the UK: initial findings from the BBC "diet trials". BMJ. 2006 3;332(7553):1309–14; Erratum in: BMJ. 2006;332(7555):1418.

84. Keys A, Menotti A, Karvonen MJ, Aravanis C, Blackburn H, Buzina R, Djordjevic BS, Dontas AS, Fidanza F, Keys MH, et al. The diet and 15-year death rate in the seven countries study. Am J Epidemiol. 1986;124(6):903–15.

85. McManus K, Antinoro L, Sacks F. A randomized controlled trial of a moderate-fat, low-energy diet compared with a low fat, low-energy diet for weight loss in overweight adults. Int J Obes Relat Metab Disord. 2001;25(10):1503–11.

86. Seccareccia F, Lanti M, Menotti A, Scanga M. Role of body mass index in the prediction of all cause mortality in over 62,000 men and women. The Italian RIFLE Pooling Project. Risk Factor and Life Expectancy. J Epidemiol Community Health. 1998;52(1):20–6.

87. Gorin AA, Phelan S, Wing RR, Hill JO. Promoting long-term weight control: does dieting consistency matter? Int J Obes Relat Metab Disord. 2004;28(2):278–81.

88. Estruch R, Martínez-González MA, Corella D, Salas-Salvadó J, Ruiz-Gutiérrez V, Covas MI, PREDIMED Study Investigators, et al. Effects of a Mediterranean-style diet on cardiovascular risk factors: a randomized trial. Ann Intern Med. 2006;145(1):1–11.

89. Vincent-Baudry S, Defoort C, Gerber M, Bernard MC, Verger P, Helal O, et al. The Medi-RIVAGE study: reduction of cardiovascular disease risk factors after a 3-mo intervention with a Mediterranean-type diet or a low-fat diet. Am J Clin Nutr. 2005;82(5):964–71.

90. Gardner CD, Kiazand A, Alhassan S, Kim S, Stafford RS, Balise RR, Kraemer HC, King AC. Comparison of the Atkins, Zone, Ornish, and LEARN diets for change in weight and related risk factors among overweight premenopausal women: the A TO Z Weight Loss Study: a randomized trial. JAMA. 2007;297(9):969–77.

91. Shai I, Schwarzfuchs D, Henkin Y, Shahar DR, Witkow S, Greenberg I, et al. Dietary Intervention Randomized Controlled Trial (DIRECT) Group. N Engl J Med2008;359:229–41. Eur Urol. 2009;55(1):249–50.

92. Beunza JJ, Toledo E, Hu FB, Bes-Rastrollo M, Serrano-Martínez M, Sánchez-Villegas A, et al. Adherence to the Mediterranean diet, long-term weight change, and incident overweight or obesity: the Seguimiento Universidad de Navarra (SUN) cohort. Am J Clin Nutr. 2010;92(6):1484–93.

93. Mendez MA, Popkin BM, Jakszyn P, Berenguer A, Tormo MJ, Sanchéz MJ, et al. Adherence to a Mediterranean diet is associated with reduced 3-year incidence of obesity. J Nutr. 2006;136(11):2934–8.

94. Shubair MM, McColl RS, Hanning RM. Mediterranean dietary components and body mass index in adults: the peel nutrition and heart health survey. Chronic Dis Can. 2005 Spring-Summer;26(2–3):43–51.

95. Panagiotakos DB, Chrysohoou C, Pitsavos C, Stefanadis C. Association between the prevalence of obesity and adherence to the Mediterranean diet: the ATTICA study. Nutrition. 2006;22(5):449–56.

96. Panagiotakos DB, Pitsavos C, Skoumas Y, Stefanadis C. The association between food patterns and the metabolic syndrome using principal components analysis: The ATTICA Study. J Am Diet Assoc. 2007;107(6):979–87; quiz 997.

97. Schröder H, Marrugat J, Vila J, Covas MI, Elosua R. Adherence to the traditional mediterranean diet is inversely associated with body mass index and obesity in a Spanish population. J Nutr. 2004;134(12):3355–61.

98. Goulet J, Lamarche B, Nadeau G, Lemieux S. Effect of a nutritional intervention promoting the Mediterranean food pattern on plasma lipids, lipoproteins and body weight in healthy French-Canadian women. Atherosclerosis. 2003;170(1):115–24.

99. Bautista-Castaño I, Doreste J, Serra-Majem L. Effectiveness of interventions in the prevention of childhood obesity. Eur J Epidemiol. 2004;19(7):617–22.

100. Esposito K, Marfella R, Ciotola M, Di Palo C, Giugliano F, Giugliano G, D'Armiento M, D'Andrea F, Giugliano D. Effect of a mediterranean-style diet on endothelial dysfunction and markers of vascular inflammation in the metabolic syndrome: a randomized trial. JAMA. 2004;292(12):1440–6.

101. Toobert DJ, Glasgow RE, Strycker LA, Barrera Jr M, Radcliffe JL, Wander RC, Bagdade JD. Biologic and quality-of-life outcomes from the Mediterranean Lifestyle Program: a randomized clinical trial. Diabetes Care. 2003;26(8):2288–93.

102. Buckland G, Bach A, Serra-Majem L. Obesity and the Mediterranean diet: a systematic review of observational and intervention studies. Obes Rev. 2008;9(6):582–93.
103. Serra-Majem L, Ferro-Luzzi A, Bellizzi M, Salleras L. Nutrition policies in Mediterranean Europe. Nutr Rev. 1997;55(11 Pt 2):S42–57.
104. Ferro-Luzzi A, Sette S. The Mediterranean Diet: an attempt to define its present and past composition. Eur J Clin Nutr. 1989;43 Suppl 2:13–29.
105. Esposito K, Kastorini CM, Panagiotakos DB, Giugliano D. Mediterranean diet and weight loss: meta-analysis of randomized controlled trials. Metab Syndr Relat Disord. 2011;9(1): 1–12.
106. US Department of Health and Human Services, Centers for Disease Control and Prevention. Physical activity for everyone: physical activity and health: the benefits of physical activity. Atlanta: CDC; 2009.
107. Adachi Y, Sato C, Yamatsu K, Ito S, Adachi K, Yamagami T. A randomized controlled trial on the long-term effects of a 1-month behavioral weight control program assisted by computer tailored advice. Behav Res Ther. 2007;45(3):459–70.
108. Carels RA, Young KM, Coit C, Clayton AM, Spencer A, Hobbs M. Can following the caloric restriction recommendations from the Dietary Guidelines for Americans help individuals lose weight? Eat Behav. 2008;9(3):328–35.
109. Helsel DL, Jakicic JM, Otto AD. Comparison of techniques for self-monitoring eating and exercise behaviors on weight loss in a correspondence-based intervention. J Am Diet Assoc. 2007;107(10):1807–10.
110. Butryn ML, Phelan S, Hill JO, Wing RR. Consistent self-monitoring of weight: a key component of successful weight loss maintenance. Obesity (Silver Spring). 2007;15(12):3091–6.
111. Wing RR, Tate DF, Gorin AA, Raynor HA, Fava JL. A self-regulation program for maintenance of weight loss. N Engl J Med. 2006;355(15):1563–71.
112. Abid A, Galuska D, Khan LK, Gillespie C, Ford ES, Serdula MK. Are healthcare professionals advising obese patients to lose weight? A trend analysis. MedGenMed. 2005;7(4):10.
113. Ma J, Xiao L, Stafford RS. Adult obesity and office-based quality of care in the United States. Obesity (Silver Spring). 2009;17(5):1077–85.
114. Centers for Disease Control and Prevention (CDC). Children and teens told by doctors that they were overweight—United States, 1999-2002. MMWR Morb Mortal Wkly Rep. 2005;54(34):848–9.
115. Johnson F, Cooke L, Croker H, Wardle J. Changing perceptions of weight in Great Britain: comparison of two population surveys. BMJ. 2008;337:a494.
116. Reedy J, Mitrou PN, Krebs-Smith SM, Wirfält E, Flood A, Kipnis V, Leitzmann M, Mouw T, Hollenbeck A, Schatzkin A, Subar AF. Index-based dietary patterns and risk of colorectal cancer: the NIH-AARP Diet and Health Study. Am J Epidemiol. 2008;168(1):38–48.
117. Wendel-Vos GC, Schuit AJ, Feskens EJ, Boshuizen HC, Verschuren WM, Saris WH, Kromhout D. Physical activity and stroke. A meta-analysis of observational data. Int J Epidemiol. 2004;33(4):787–98.
118. Evenson KR, Rosamond WD, Cai J, Toole JF, Hutchinson RG, Shahar E, Folsom AR. Physical activity and ischemic stroke risk. The atherosclerosis risk in communities study. Stroke. 1999;30(7):1333–9.
119. Hu FB, Stampfer MJ, Colditz GA, Ascherio A, Rexrode KM, Willett WC, Manson JE. Physical activity and risk of stroke in women. JAMA. 2000;283(22):2961–7.
120. Tanasescu M, Leitzmann MF, Rimm EB, Willett WC, Stampfer MJ, Hu FB. Exercise type and intensity in relation to coronary heart disease in men. JAMA. 2002;288(16):1994–2000.
121. Shaw K, Gennat H, O'Rourke P, Del Mar C. Exercise for overweight or obesity. Cochrane Database Syst Rev. 2006;(4):CD003817.
122. Pate RR, Pratt M, Blair SN, Haskell WL, Macera CA, Bouchard C, et al. Physical activity and public health. A recommendation from the Centers for Disease Control and Prevention and the American College of Sports Medicine. JAMA. 1995;273(5):402–7.
123. Yusuf S, Hawken S, Ounpuu S, Dans T, Avezum A, Lanas F, INTERHEART Study Investigators, et al. Effect of potentially modifiable risk factors associated with myocardial

infarction in 52 countries (the INTERHEART study): case-control study. Lancet. 2004;364(9438): 937–52.

124. Lee CD, Folsom AR, Blair SN. Physical activity and stroke risk: a meta-analysis. Stroke. 2003;34(10):2475–81.

125. US Department of Health and Human Services, Centers for Disease Control and Prevention. Physical activity for everyone: physical activity and health: the benefits of physical activity. Atlanta: CDC; 2009.

126. American Heart Association (AHA). http://circ.ahajournals.org/content/123/4/e18.full.pdf. Accessed May 27, 2011.

127. Pleis JR, Lucas JW. Summary health statistics for U.S. adults: National Health Interview Survey, 2007. Vital Health Stat 10. 2009;(240):1–159.

128. Troiano RP, Berrigan D, Dodd KW, Mâsse LC, Tilert T, McDowell M. Physical activity in the United States measured by accelerometer. Med Sci Sports Exerc. 2008;40(1):181–8.

129. Eaton DK, Kann L, Kinchen S, Shanklin S, Ross J, Hawkins J, et al.; Centers for Disease Control and Prevention (CDC). Youth risk behavior surveillance–United States, 2007. MMWR Surveill Summ. 2008;57(4):1–131.

130. Dietz WH, Gortmaker SL. Preventing obesity in children and adolescents. Annu Rev Public Health. 2001;22:337–53.

131. McDonald NC. Active transportation to school: trends among U.S. schoolchildren, 1969-2001. Am J Prev Med. 2007;32(6):509–16.

132. Dunstan DW, Barr EL, Healy GN, Salmon J, Shaw JE, Balkau B, et al. Television viewing time and mortality: the Australian Diabetes, Obesity and Lifestyle Study (AusDiab). Circulation. 2010;121(3):384–91.

133. Levine JA, Schleusner SJ, Jensen MD. Energy expenditure of nonexercise activity. Am J Clin Nutr. 2000;72(6):1451–4.

134. Centers for Medicare and Medicaid Services. http://www.cms.gov/apps/media/press/release.asp?Counter=4189&intNumPerPage=10&checkDate=&checkKey=&srchType=1&numDays=3500&sr (29 Nov 2011 press release). Accessed 1 Dec 2011.

135. Centers for Medicare and Medicaid Services. Decision summary. http://www.cms.gov/medi-care-coverage-database/details/nca-decision-memo.aspx?&NcaName=Intensive%20Behavioral%20Therapy%20for%20Obesity&bc=ACAAAAAAIAAA&NCAId=253. Accessed 1 Dec 2011.

Part IV
Macronutrients

Chapter 10
Macronutrients in an Adherence Score: Carbohydrates, Proteins, Fats, and Alcohol

Keywords Macronutrient classes • Carbohydrates • Proteins • Fats • Alcohol

The categories used in calculating a Mediterranean diet adherence score contain foods comprised of nutrients from the three macronutrient classes—carbohydrates, proteins, and fats—as well as from the unique subclass, alcohol. A review of each of these classes follows. Information on their nomenclature and the health effects of their constituent nutrients is provided to strengthen understanding of basic nutrition and why certain foods are emphasized in a MedDiet. Although educating patients about a MedDiet does not necessarily require a provider to master the complexities of human nutrition, having a working understanding of major concepts is useful.

E. Zacharias, *The Mediterranean Diet: A Clinician's Guide for Patient Care*, 103
DOI 10.1007/978-1-4614-3326-2_10, © Springer Science+Business Media, LLC 2012

Chapter 11
Fats and Oils

Keywords Mediterranean diet • Saturated fatty acid • Monounsaturated fatty acid • Polyunsaturated fatty acid • Triacylglycerols • Triglycerides • Phospholipids • Cholesterol • Lipoproteins

Understanding the structure, function, nomenclature, and clinical effects of fats is necessary when discussing a Mediterranean diet with patients. The most important concept regarding fats is that they can vary greatly in their health effects on the human body. In the past, knowledge that avoidance of some fats could reduce heart disease led to overly general recommendations to avoid all fats, irrespective of type. As a result of advances in understanding the benefits of consuming so-called healthy fats, advice to avoid all types of fats as a strategy for health is now rare in the medical literature. For example, the American Heart Association (AHA), a former advocate for aggressive restriction of all fats, no longer advises this strategy. The AHA dietary guidelines recognize that, consistent with a MedDiet, obtaining up to 35% of all calories from healthy unsaturated fatty acids while avoiding *trans*-fats and minimizing saturated fatty acids (SFAs) is an effective coronary heart disease preventive dietary strategy [1, 2].

All dietary fats provide nine calories of energy per gram. Learning the nomenclature is more than an academic exercise as fats are frequently named by their scientific name in both professional and lay writings, often with the assumption that the reader understands their class, structure, and consequent function in the body. This foundation of understanding will help prevent the avoidable confusion regarding fat consumption that occurred in the 1980s and 1990s when it was a commonplace strategy to tell patients, based on the fact that some fats are indeed bad for health,

E. Zacharias, *The Mediterranean Diet: A Clinician's Guide for Patient Care*,
DOI 10.1007/978-1-4614-3326-2_11, © Springer Science+Business Media, LLC 2012

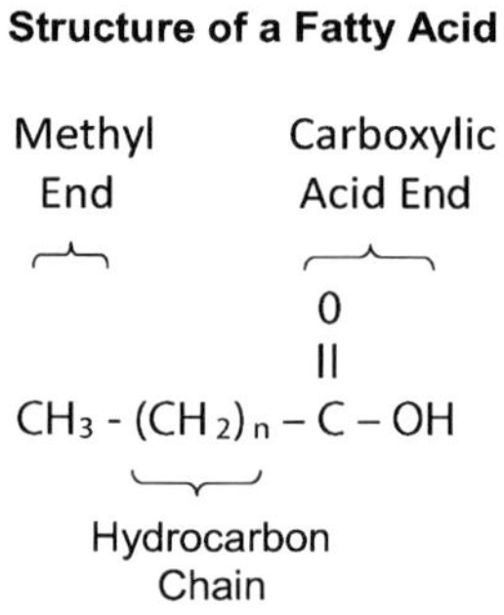

Fig. 11.1 Basic fatty acid   **Structure of a Fatty Acid**

Methyl   Carboxylic
End   Acid End

$$CH_3 - (CH_2)_n - C - OH$$

with the O double-bonded ($||$) to C

Hydrocarbon
Chain

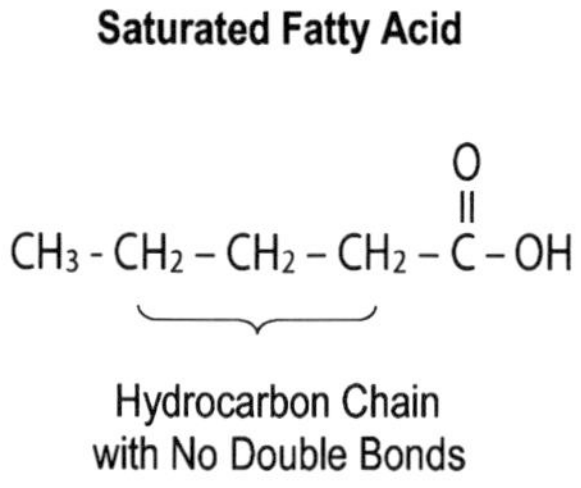

Fig. 11.2 Saturated fatty acid   **Saturated Fatty Acid**

$$CH_3 - CH_2 - CH_2 - CH_2 - C - OH$$

with the O double-bonded ($||$) to C

Hydrocarbon Chain
with No Double Bonds

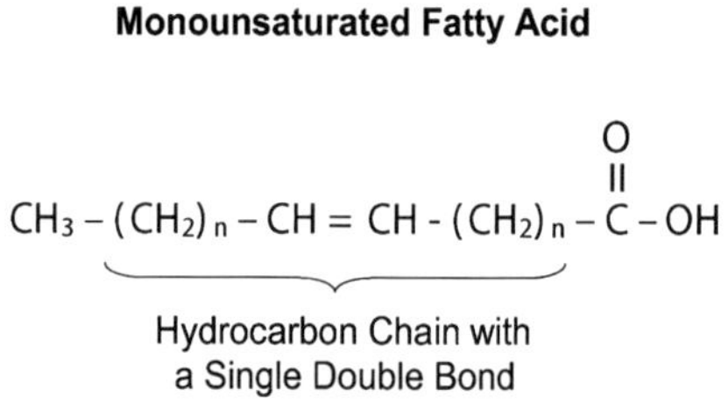

Fig. 11.3 Monounsaturated fatty acid   **Monounsaturated Fatty Acid**

$$CH_3 - (CH_2)_n - CH = CH - (CH_2)_n - C - OH$$

with the O double-bonded ($||$) to C

Hydrocarbon Chain with
a Single Double Bond

that they should avoid all fats to optimize their health. If patients seek more information from more professionally oriented publications, this knowledge will also help them to avoid confusion or frustration.

The nomenclature of dietary fats follows.

Fatty Acids

Fatty acids (FA) are the most simple lipid form. They are comprised of a hydrocarbon chain with a carboxylic acid group on one end (Fig. 11.1).

If the hydrocarbon chain of a fatty acid contains no double bonds, then the fatty acid is referred to as a SFA (Fig. 11.2). SFAs are solid at room temperature.

If the hydrocarbon chain of a fatty acid contains a single carbon-to-carbon double bond, then it is referred to as a monounsaturated fatty acid (MUFA) (Fig. 11.3). MUFAs are liquid, oils, at room temperature.

Fig. 11.4 Polyunsaturated
fatty acid

Polyunsaturated Fatty Acid

$$CH_3 - (CH_2)_n - CH = CH - (CH_2)_n - CH = CH - (CH_2)_n - \overset{\overset{\textstyle O}{\|}}{C} - OH$$

Hydrocarbon Chain with
Two or More Double Bonds

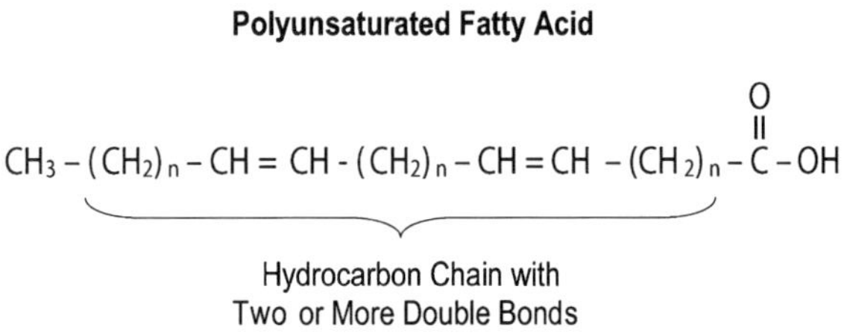

Fig. 11.5 *Cis*-conformation

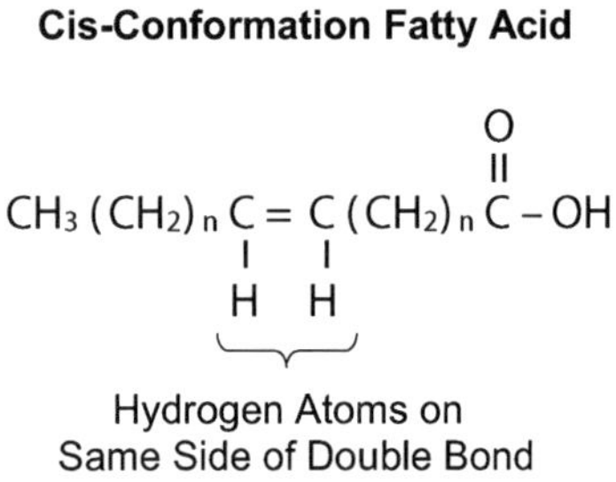

Cis-Conformation Fatty Acid

$$CH_3 (CH_2)_n \underset{\overset{|}{H}}{C} = \underset{\overset{|}{H}}{C} (CH_2)_n \overset{\overset{\textstyle O}{\|}}{C} - OH$$

Hydrogen Atoms on
Same Side of Double Bond

Fig. 11.6 *Trans*-conformation

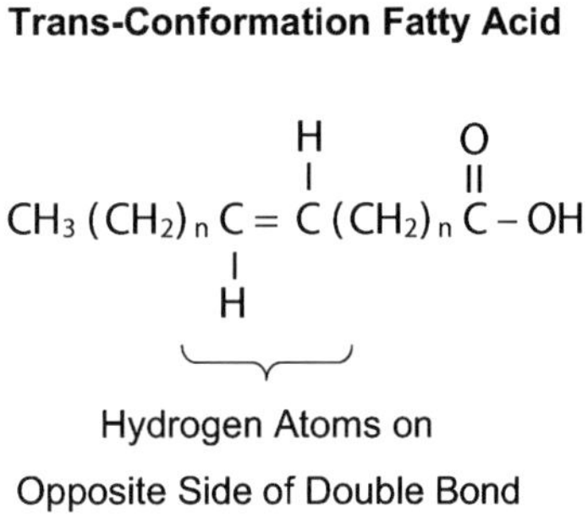

Trans-Conformation Fatty Acid

$$CH_3 (CH_2)_n \underset{\overset{|}{H}}{\overset{\overset{\textstyle H}{|}}{C}} = C (CH_2)_n \overset{\overset{\textstyle O}{\|}}{C} - OH$$

Hydrogen Atoms on
Opposite Side of Double Bond

If the hydrocarbon chain of a fatty acid contains two or more carbon-to-carbon double bonds, then it is referred to as a polyunsaturated fatty acid (PUFA) (Fig. 11.4). PUFAs are liquid, oils, at room temperature.

The physical conformation of fatty acids is also described in nomenclature. *Cis*-conformation at a double bond means that the hydrogen atoms bonded to each of the carbons of the double bond are physically located on the same side (Fig. 11.5). This is the conformation of the overwhelming preponderance of naturally occurring fatty acids. By convention, it is implied that a fatty acid is in the *cis*-conformation unless otherwise noted.

Trans-conformation at a double bond means that the hydrogen atoms bonded to each of the carbons of the double bond are physically located on opposite sides (Fig. 11.6). Although this conformation is found in trace quantities in some animal fats, the overwhelming preponderance of *trans*-conformation fatty acids in the diet is created by the processed food industry via partial hydrogenation. Information about the detrimental health effects of *trans*-fatty acids is contained in this chapter.

Advanced Nomenclature

Fats are frequently referred to by their category, formula, carbon-to-double-bonds ratio, omega system (n-system), delta system, systematic name, and common name. The formula method for referring to a fatty acid notes the hydrocarbon length and double bond position, if present, between the methyl and carboxyl ends (Fig. 11.7a). Simple notation method lists the number of carbons present followed by the number of double bonds (Fig. 11.7b). All SFAs will be represented with the number zero following the number of carbon atoms, as they have no double bonds. All MUFAs will have the number one following the number of carbon atoms, as they always have exactly one double bond. All PUFAs will have the number two or a greater number following the number of carbon atoms, as they always have two or more double bonds.

Two additional methods used for referring to fatty acids are the Omega notation (ω-) and the Delta notation (Δ-) (Fig. 11.7c). Omega notation denotes the position of the first carbon that contains a double bond counting from the methyl end of the fatty acid. If, for example, the position of the first carbon containing a double bond counting from the methyl end were located at the sixth position, then the Omega notation would be ω-6. By convention, the letter "n-" is frequently substituted for the omega symbol so that ω-6 could also be written as n-6. These are synonyms. One might see the identical fatty acids referred to as "omega-3 fatty acids," "ω-3 fatty acids," or "n-3 fatty acids" in different articles. The Omega notation is limited in that it exclusively names the position of the first double bond in a fatty acid irrespective of the presence of additional double bonds. The Delta notation names the position of all double bonds in a fatty acid. In contrast to Omega notation, the Delta notation counts location starting from the carboxyl end and names all double bonds present as superscripts on the delta symbol. The Delta and Omega notation systems are occasionally used jointly when naming fatty acids.

Lastly, fatty acids are referred to by their common name. This name is often related to a fatty acid's chemical structure, source in nature, or chemical properties. A reference table applying the previously outlined nomenclature to the most common and important dietary fatty acids follows (Table 11.1).

There are additional fats and lipids commonly encountered in the popular and medical literature on nutrition:

Triacylglycerols

Triacylglycerols (TAG), also called triglycerides, are comprised of three fatty acids attached to a molecule of glycerol (Fig. 11.8). The three fatty acids of TAGs can be any combination of SFAs, MUFAs, and PUFAs. The TAGs are generally solid at room temperature if they contain predominately SFA and generally liquid if predominately MUFA and/or PUFA. TAG are both the main form of fats in the diet and the main storage form of fats in the body.

Three Types of Nomenclature

Formula Notation:

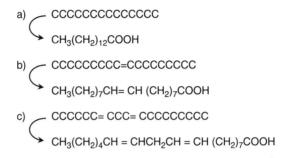

a) CCCCCCCCCCCCCC

$CH_3(CH_2)_{12}COOH$

b) CCCCCCCCC=CCCCCCCCC

$CH_3(CH_2)_7CH= CH (CH_2)_7COOH$

c) CCCCCC= CCC= CCCCCCCCC

$CH_3(CH_2)_4CH = CHCH_2CH = CH (CH_2)_7COOH$

Simple Notation:

a)   14:0

b)   18:1

c)   18:2

Omega Notation and Delta Notation:

a) Not applicable since no double bonds

b) **Omega**   **Delta**
carbon   carbon
count from   ω-9   Δ9   count from
methyl end ──→1   2-8   9 \|/ 9 2-8   1 ←── carboxyl end
                     $CH_3(CH_2)_7$ CH = CH $(CH_2)_7$ COOH

Omega Notation	Delta Notation	Combined
18:1 ω-9	18:1 Δ9	18:1 Δ9 (ω-9)
or, 18:1 n-9		18:1 Δ9 (n-9)

c)   ω-6   Δ12   Δ9
       ──→1   2-5   6 \|/12 11 10 / 9   2 -8   1←──
                  $CH_3(CH_2)_4$ CH =CHCH_2CH = CH $(CH_2)_7$ COOH

Omega Notation	Delta Notation	Combined
18:2 ω-6	18:2 Δ9,12	18:2 Δ9,12 (ω-6)
or, 18:2 n-6		18:2 Δ9,12 (n-6)

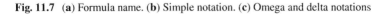

Fig. 11.7 (**a**) Formula name. (**b**) Simple notation. (**c**) Omega and delta notations

Table 11.1 Common dietary fatty acids

Common name	Notation	Structure
Saturated fatty acids (SFAs)		
Lauric	12:0	$CH_3(CH_2)_{10}COOH$
Myristic	14:0	$CH_3(CH_2)_{12}COOH$
Palmitic	16:0	$CH_3(CH_2)_{14}COOH$
Stearic	18:0	$CH_3(CH_2)_{16}COOH$
Monounsaturated fatty acids (MUFAs)		
Palmitoleic	$16:1\Delta^9$ (n-7)	$CH_3(CH_2)_5CH=CH(CH_2)_7COOH$
Oleic	$18:1\Delta^9$ (n-9)	$CH_3(CH_2)_7CH=CH(CH_2)_7COOH$
Polyunsaturated fatty acids (PUFAs)t		
Linoleic	$18:2\Delta^{9,12}$ (n-6)	$CH_3(CH_2)_4CH=CHCH_2CH=CH(CH_2)_7COOH$
Alpha-linolenic	$18:3\Delta^{9,12,15}$ (n-3)	$CH_3(CH_2CH=CH_2)_3(CH_2)_7COOH$
Arachidonic	$20:4\Delta^{5,8,11,14}$ (n-6)	$CH_3(CH_2)_4(CH=CHCH_2)_4(CH_2)_7COOH$
Eicosapentaenoic (EPA)	$20:5\Delta^{5,8,11,14,17}$ (n-3)	$CH_3(CH_2CH=CH)_5(CH_2)_3COOH$
Docosahexaenoic (DHA)	$22:6\Delta^{4,7,10,13,16,19}$ (n-3)	$CH_3(CH_2CH=CH)_6(CH_2)_2COOH$

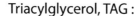

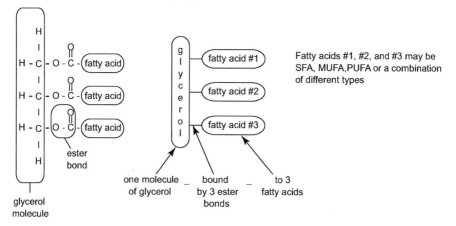

Fig. 11.8 Triacylglycerol

Phospholipids

Phospholipids have a nearly identical structure to TAGs, but the third fatty acid bound to glycerol is replaced with a phosphate bound to a hydrophilic polar head group (Fig. 11.9).

Cholesterol

Cholesterol contains a four-ring core with an attached hydroxyl group and carbon side chain (Fig. 11.10). The hydroxyl group may bind to a fatty acid via an ester bond to form a cholesterol ester.

Phospholipid

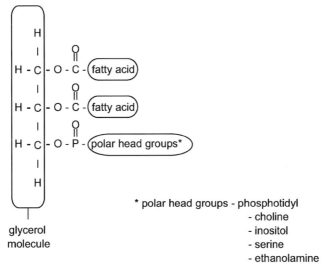

* polar head groups - phosphotidyl
- choline
- inositol
- serine
- ethanolamine

Fig. 11.9 Phospholipids

Lipoproteins

Relative to the aforementioned lipids, lipoproteins are enormous, complex compounds (Fig. 11.11). They are comprised of a core of hydrophobic cholesterol esters and triglycerides with a surface of hydrophilic apolipoproteins, phospholipids, and cholesterol. Their chief role is to transport TAGs and cholesterol throughout the body. Biological properties and health effects of lipoproteins vary depending on their size and relative amounts and types of surface apolipoproteins. Lipoproteins tend to be of greater size and lesser density the more fat relative to protein that they contain.

The surfaces of the different lipoproteins contain different types, relative amounts, and combinations of apolipoproteins. These include types A-I, A-II, A-IV, B 100, B 48, C-I, C-II, C-III, D, E, H, J, L 1-6, M, and (a). Although these apolipoproteins will be referred to on occasion in the medical literature on health effects of diet, a detailed discussion of their myriad functions is beyond the scope of this book.

A simplified summary of the two most highly studied lipoproteins, low-density lipoprotein (LDL) and high-density lipoprotein (HDL) can be shared with patients. LDL carries cholesterol to the tissues, and higher levels of LDL are strongly associated with higher levels of cardiovascular disease (CVD) [3]. LDL is commonly referred to as "the bad cholesterol." HDL is the major carrier of cholesterol from the tissues to the liver for processing and excretion in the bile. The process performed by HDL can be described as reverse cholesterol transport, and so HDL is commonly referred to as "the good cholesterol." Higher levels of HDL are strongly associated with reduced rates of CVD [4]. When looking at the recommended fats in a MedDiet, understanding their effects on LDL and HDL illuminates why some fats are

Cholesterol

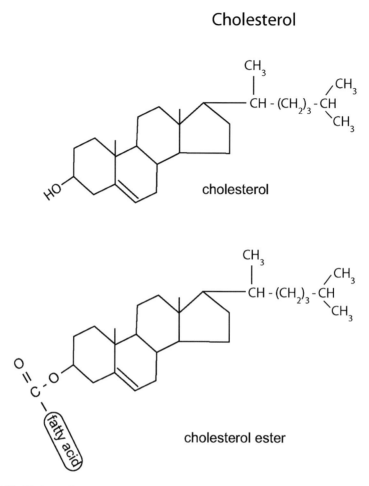

Fig. 11.10 Cholesterol

encouraged and others are to be avoided. Dietary SFA increases LDL, *trans*-FA increase LDL and decrease HDL, and MUFA and PUFA decrease LDL and raise HDL [5]. Due to these unfavorable effects on lipoproteins, SFA should be restricted and *trans*-FA completely avoided. The favorable lipoprotein effects of MUFA and PUFA are one of several reasons their consumption is encouraged.

Biology and Health Effects

Once the basic nomenclature of fats and lipids is understood, a discussion with patients on their practical health effects may be started. The first category to start with can be SFAs.

Lipoprotein

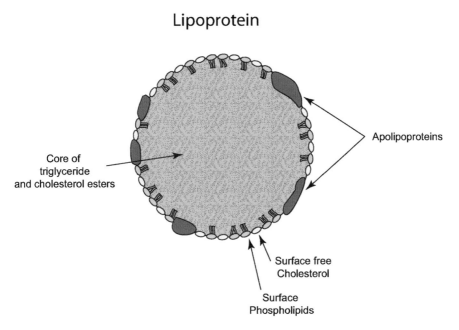

Core of
triglyceride
and cholesterol esters

Apolipoproteins

Surface free
Cholesterol

Surface
Phospholipids

Fig. 11.11 Lipoprotein

SFA

The SFAs as an overall class are strongly associated with increased heart disease, strokes, and diabetes, and their consumption is restricted to low levels in a MedDiet. There are four important dietary SFAs: lauric, myristic, palmitic, and stearic. Of the four, only stearic acid is not strongly associated with biological actions proven to increase disease. In a comprehensive analysis of published major studies assessing health effects of SFAs on a combined total of more than 340,000 subjects, the Dietary Guidelines for Americans Advisory Committee 2010 reached the following conclusions: "Strong evidence indicates that dietary SFAs are positively associated with intermediate markers and end-point health outcomes for two distinct metabolic pathways: (1) increased serum total cholesterol and LDL cholesterol and increased risk of CVD, and, (2) increased risk of type 2 diabetes (T2D). Conversely, decreased SFA intake improves measures of both CVD and T2D risk. The evidence shows that a 5% energy decrease in SFA, replaced by MUFA or PUFA decreases risk of CVD and T2D in healthy adults and improved insulin responsiveness in insulin resistant and T2D subjects" [5]. Numerous other researchers also recommend that to improve health outcomes, people should reduce SFA consumption and replace SFA with unsaturated fatty acids [6–18]. Fats and their SFA content are shown in Table 11.2.

Table 11.2 Fatty acid content of dietary fats

Fatty acid content of dietary fats per 100 g of fat

Fat source	Saturated fatty acids	Unsaturated fatty acids				
	Total SFA	Total MUFA	Total PUFA	Linoleic (n-6)	Alpha-linolenic (n-3)	EPH and DHA and DPA (n-3)
Almond oil	8.2	69.9	17.4	17.4	0	0
Avocado oil	11.6	70.5	13.5	12.6	1.0	0
Beef tallow	49.8	41.8	4.0	3.1	0.6	0
Butter	51.4	21.0	3.0	2.7	0.3	0
Canola oil	7.1	58.9	29.6	20.3	9.3	0
Cocoa butter	59.7	32.9	3	2.8	0.1	0
Coconut oil	86.5	5.8	1.8	1.8	0	0
Corn oil	12.9	27.6	54.7	53.5	1.2	0
Flaxseed oil	9.4	20.2	66	12.7	53.3	0
Grapeseed oil	9.6	16.1	69.9	69.6	0.1	0
Hazelnut oil	7.4	78	10.2	10.1	0	0
Herring oil	21.3	56.6	15.6	1.1	0.8	11.1
Lard	39.2	45.1	11.2	10.2	1	0
Olive oil	13.5	73.7	8.5	7.9	0.6	0
Palm oil	49.3	37	9.3	9.1	0.2	0
Palm kernel oil	81.5	11.4	1.6	1.6	0	0
Pistachio oil	13.8	49.3	32.5	13.2	0	0
Peanut oil	16.9	46.2	32	32	0	0
Safflower oil	6.2	14.4	74.6	74.6	0	0
Salmon oil	19.9	29.0	40.3	1.5	1.1	34.2
Sesame oil	14.2	39.7	41.7	41.3	0.3	0
Soybean oil	14.4	23.3	57.9	51	6.8	0
Walnut oil	9.1	22.8	63.3	52.9	10.4	0

Adapted from Position of the American Dietetic Association and Dietitians of Canada: dietary fatty acids. *J Am Dietetic Assoc.* 2007. http://www.nal.usda.gov/fnic/foodcomp/search

MUFA

The next category to discuss is the MUFAs. The MUFA, palmitoleic and oleic acid, are an important part of a MedDiet, and they are associated with numerous favorable health outcomes. The most current systematic review of published major studies assessing the health effects of MUFA on health outcomes comes from the DGAC, 2010, which reached the following conclusion: "Strong evidence indicates that dietary MUFA are associated with improved blood lipids related to both CVD and T2D, when they are a replacement for dietary SFA. The evidence shows that 5% energy replacement of SFA with MUFA decreases intermediate markers and the risk of CVD and T2D in healthy adults and improves insulin responsiveness in T2D subjects." Other quality studies also support the recommendation to consume MUFA as a part of a healthy diet [19–25]. Fats and their MUFA content are given in Table 11.2.

Trans-MUFA

Trans-MUFAs are a special case. Although there are trace amounts of the *trans*-fatty acids vaccenic acid in some animal fats, the overwhelming majority of them in the diet are industrially produced by partial hydrogenation of oils. *Trans*-fatty acids are associated with increased LDL-cholesterol, decreased HDL-cholesterol, and increased overall CVD. A meta-analysis of multiple prospective trials showed a 23% increase in CHD risk for each 2% increase in calories from *trans*-fats [26]. In a report of effects of modifiable risk factors, higher consumption of *trans*-fats was estimated to account for 82,000 annual, preventable deaths [27]. The most recent DGAC, 2010 advises avoidance of all *trans*-fatty acids [5].

PUFA

The next category to discuss is the PUFAs. The PUFAs are an important part of a MedDiet. They are associated with numerous favorable health outcomes.

The most current systematic review of published studies assessing the health effects of PUFA on health outcomes comes from the DGAC, 2010: "strong and consistent evidence indicates that dietary n-6 PUFA are associated with improved blood lipids related to CVD, in particular when PUFA is a replacement for dietary SFA or *trans*-fatty acids. Evidence shows that energy replacement of SFA with PUFA decreases total cholesterol, LDL-cholesterol and triglycerides, as well as numerous markers of inflammation. PUFA intake significantly decreases risk of CVD and has also been shown to decrease the risk of T2D" [5]. In the studies reviewed for the DGAC, 2010, there was not a significant difference between the n-6 fatty acid, linoleic acid (LA), and the n-3 fatty acid, alpha-linolenic acid (ALA), in beneficial effects when substituted for SFA [5, 28, 29]. In independent analysis of 11 studies with a combined total of more than 340,000 individuals, replacement of SFA with PUFA was determined to reduce CHD risk in a linear and continuous fashion [25].

The complexity of the PUFAs and their metabolites can be a source of confusion. The frequent referencing of "omega-3's" and "fish oil" in the popular press warrants spending time with patients to teach them about this important class of fats. The two main PUFAs are linoleic acid (LA), which is an omega-6 FA, and ALA, which is an omega-3 FA. These two PUFAs are known as essential FA because they must be obtained from dietary sources. Humans are incapable of synthesizing them. Through the actions of desaturation and elongation enzymes, both LA and ALA serve as precursors for other important fatty acids. These synthetic pathways are shown in Fig. 11.12. When reviewing these pathways, note that ALA can serve as a precursor for the frequently discussed and written about omega-3 FA contained in fish oils, eicosapentaenoic acid (EPA) (20:5, n-3) and docosahexaenoic acid (DHA) (22:6, n-3). The conversion of ALA to EPA and DHA has been reported to occur at a rate of 0–20% amount depending on as yet incompletely understood variables [30]. The DGAC, 2010 determined there is insufficient evidence as to whether one variable, the presence of n-6 FA, competitively inhibits this conversion process. Prostaglandins and leukotrienes derived from the omega-3 FA tend to exhibit favorable vascular effects of an anti-inflammatory, antiaggretory, and vasodilatory nature. Prostaglandins and leukotrienes derived from omega-6 FA often have the opposite effects. The clinical significance of these differences is not yet known.

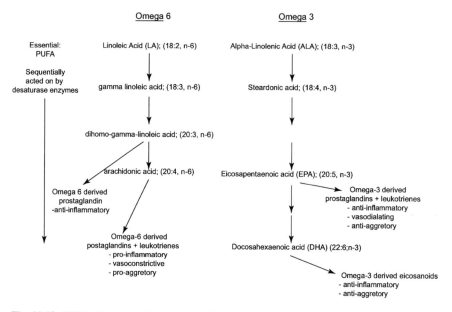

Fig. 11.12 PUFA: the omega-6 and omega-3 fatty acids

Table 11.3 Common sources of omega three fatty acids. http://www.nal.usda.gov/fnic/foodcomp/search

Source	Total n-3s	Alpha-linolenic	EPA and DHA and DPA
Flaxseed oil	53.3	53.3	0
Fish oil, salmon oil	35.3	1.06	34.24
Fish oil, sardine oil	24.1	1.33	22.77
Milled flax seeds	22.81	22.81	0
Fish oil, herring oil	11.9	0.8	11.1
Walnut oil	10.4	10.4	0
Canola oil	9.3	9.3	0
Soy bean oil	6.8	6.8	0
Wild Atlantic salmon	2.59	0.38	2.21
Canned anchovies	2.12	0.02	2.10
Walnuts	2.0	2.0	0
Canned sardines	1.48	0.50	0.98
Mackerel	1.42	0.11	1.31
Soy beans	1.33	1.33	0
Wild trout, rainbow	1.19	0.19	1.0
Pecans	0.99	0.99	0
Tuna, canned white	0.95	0.07	0.88
Sea bass	0.86	0	0.86
Shrimp	0.12	0.01	0.11

There are purported health benefits to the n-3 fatty acids, and their consumption, particularly those obtained from fish, has been a focus of intense research over the past several years. The most recent DGAC, 2010 reviewed 28 studies published since 2004 and reached the following conclusion, "Moderate evidence shows that consumption of two servings of seafood per week, which provides an average of 250 mg per day of long-chain n-3 FA, is associated with reduced cardiac mortality from CHD as well as sudden death in persons with CVD" [5]. Sources of omega-3 fatty acids are noted in Table 11.3.

Special Focus: How Safe Is Seafood to Eat?

Seafood can be an excellent source for the omega-3 fatty acids EPA and DHA (Table 11.3) and serve as a healthy source for protein. Academic nutritionists frequently create a separate, favorable category for seafood when calculating a MedDiet-AS. However, seafood also may be contaminated with methyl mercury and organic pollutants and may be harvested in ways that are either unsustainable or environmentally destructive. In its 2010 guidelines, the DGAC reviewed the published evidence for risks vs. benefits for seafood consumption and reached the following conclusion, "Moderate, consistent evidence shows that health benefits derived from the consumption of a variety of cooked seafood in the US in amounts recommended by the Committee (two servings per week) outweigh the risks

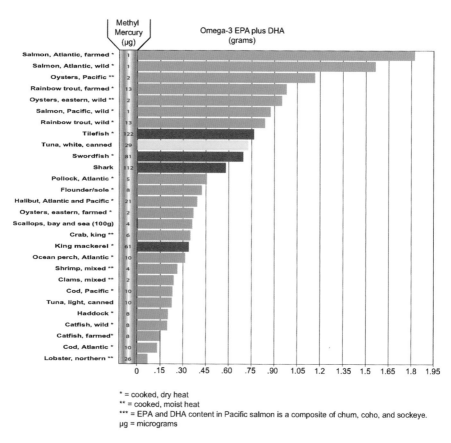

Fig. 11.13 Omega 3 and mercury. Modified from ref. [31]

associated with methyl mercury and persistent organic pollutants exposure. Overall, consumers can safely eat at least 12 oz (340 g) of a variety of cooked seafood per week, provided they pay attention to local seafood advisories and limit their intake of large, predatory fish. Women who may become or who are pregnant, nursing mothers, and children ages 12 and younger can safely consume a variety of cooked seafood in amounts recommended by this Committee, while following Federal and local advisories" [5]. Figure 11.13 shows the amounts of EPA plus DHA and methyl mercury content of seafood [31].

A review of the environmental impacts of the world's seafood harvesting and farming practices is outside the scope of this book. Patients interested in learning more about this topic may be directed to the Monterey Bay Aquarium, Natural Resources Defense Council, and Environmental Defense Fund, which maintain seafood guides on their Web sites [32–34].

Fatty Acid Contents of Various Foods

Table 11.2 lists the percentages of the different fatty acids in the most common dietary fats.

Cholesterol

Understanding cholesterol sources and metabolism is important because it plays a key role in the development of CVD (see Chap. 4 for a review of atherogenesis). All dietary sources of cholesterol are of animal origin. Figure 11.14 lists the cholesterol content of some common foods.

A fact that surprises many of my patients is that the majority of cholesterol in the body does not come from the diet at all, but it is synthesized by cells in the liver and other tissues. In fact, if a diet is completely devoid of any cholesterol whatsoever, such as in a vegan diet, the cells of the body are still capable of synthesizing all of the cholesterol required for structural and biochemical precursor purposes. Thus, cholesterol is not an essential nutrient (one that must be obtained from the diet). When carried as part of LDL, cholesterol is transported to the tissues in a fashion that has been demonstrated to increase CVD. A linear relationship exists between level of LDL-carried cholesterol and risk of CHD [35]. When carried as part of HDL, cholesterol is removed from the tissues and transported to the liver for excretion in a fashion that has been demonstrated to decrease CVD.

In a review of 14 major studies, consumption of cholesterol in an amount equivalent to greater than seven whole eggs per week was strongly associated with increased risk for CVD. However, at smaller amounts, there was not a clear association with increased risk except in individuals with T2D [5]. Numerous studies have demonstrated that SFA consumption and *trans*-FA consumption have a larger effect on raising LDL-cholesterol and consequent increased CVD risk than consumption of cholesterol itself [36–45]. As noted earlier, the MUFA and PUFA have been associated with reductions in levels of LDL and increases in HDL with consequent decreased CVD.

In summary, small amounts of dietary cholesterol have not been clearly demonstrated to increase CVD except for in individuals with T2D. However, higher levels of cholesterol intake are associated with increased CVD. Increased dietary SFA and any level of *trans*-FA consumption increase LDL and CVD. Increased dietary MUFA and PUFA decrease LDL, increase HDL, and reduce CVD.

Total Cholesterol Content in 100 gm of Common Foods

Food (100 gm)	Cholesterol Content (gm)
Whole Eggs	4.2
Butter	2.4
Pork Sausage	1.35
Cheddar Cheese	1
Chicken White Meat	0.64
Beef Steak	0.36
Whole Milk	0.32
Codfish, Halibut, Salmon	0.05
Egg Whites, All Nuts, Avocado, Legumes, and Plant Sources	0

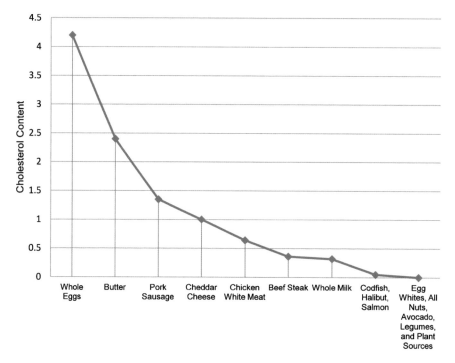

Fig. 11.14 Cholesterol in food [48]

There are three high fat foods that are often inquired about in discussions with patients on dietary fats. These are chocolate, nuts, and olive oil.

Chocolate

Although not a specifically emphasized food in a MedDiet, dark chocolate is frequently in the news when reports are published regarding its potential health effects. Certainly, the pleasure many people obtain with consuming chocolate makes it a perennially popular topic to write on in the lay press. Chocolate's chief fat-containing component is cocoa butter. This is rich in the SFA stearic acid, 18:0, which is the only SFA considered mostly neutral in its CVD effects. It also contains a moderate amount of palmitic acid, 16:0, which is considered to have adverse CVD effects. (See Table 11.2 for complete fatty acid profile of cocoa butter.) Chocolate contains the polyphenol flavonoids, a likely source for any of its health benefits. These flavonoids have favorable effects of reducing blood pressure, inflammatory markers, and LDL while raising HDL. The DGAC, 2010 concluded that, "Moderate evidence suggests that modest consumption of dark chocolate or cocoa is associated with health benefits in the form of reduced CVD risk. Potential health benefits need to be balanced with caloric intake" [5]. My conclusion is that if one enjoys dark chocolate, then consuming it in moderation is almost certainly not harmful and may have some favorable health effects. However, any extra calories obtained from chocolate should be compensated for with reduced calories from another food source.

Nuts

Nuts are often included as an individual category in the calculation of a MedDiet-AS. The most recent comprehensive review of studies published on the health effects of nuts in the DGAC, 2010 concluded, "There is moderate evidence that consumption of unsalted peanuts and tree nuts, specifically walnuts, almonds, and pistachios, in the context of a nutritionally adequate diet and when total caloric intake is held constant has a favorable impact in CVD risk factors, particularly, serum lipid levels" [5]. My conclusion is that nuts, both in whole form and as nut butters, are a convenient, flavorful, and healthy way to improve the quality of one's diet. The fat content of various nuts is listed in Table 11.4.

Olive Oil

Olive oil is a key ingredient in many of the traditional Mediterranean foods. It is also a rich source of MUFA, with 70–80% of its fatty acids being oleic acid (see Table 11.2; fatty acids). The two main categories of olive oil are virgin and refined. Virgin olive oil is extracted from the fruit exclusively by mechanical means that do

Table 11.4 Protein and fat content of nuts

Protein and fat content of nuts (per 100 g)

	Protein	SFA	MUFA	PUFA	n-3
Peanuts	25.8	6.8	24.4	15.6	0
Almonds	21.2	3.7	30.9	12.1	0
Walnuts	15.2	6.1	8.9	47.1	9.1
Pecans	9.2	6.2	40.1	21.6	1.0
Macadamia	7.9	12.1	58.9	1.5	0.2
Cashews	18.2	7.8	23.8	7.8	0.1
Pistachios	20.3	5.6	23.8	13.7	0.1
Hazelnuts	15.0	4.5	45.7	7.9	0.1

Source: www.nal.usda.gov/fric/foodcomp

not alter the oil's composition whereas the production of refined olive oils requires heat and chemical processing. Extra virgin olive oil is virgin olive oil that has been judged to be of superior flavor, mouth feel, and aroma and having a low level of acidity [46]. Olive oil is made of two components: major and minor. The major component, comprising 98% of the oil, is the TAG. The minor component, comprising approximately 2% of the oil, is the hundreds of phytochemicals in the oil with the polyphenols being the most common and most studied. Polyphenols, also an important component of dark chocolate, might have favorable cardiovascular, anti-inflammatory, and other beneficial health effects. Of note, polyphenols are mostly destroyed in the refining process so virgin olive oils have ten times or greater the polyphenol content compared to refined oils [47]. It is an open question as to whether virgin olive oil delivers health benefits from its phenols in addition to those from its high MUFA content. For now, I tell patients the health benefits from using virgin olive oil arise from the intrinsic benefits of its MUFA and possibly from its phenols as well as from the fact that when one uses virgin olive oil in cooking and flavoring foods it may be substituting for the harmful SFA and *trans*-fats found in butter, shortening, margarine, and animal fats. The fact that olive oil has a delicious flavor and is used in many of the best Mediterranean dishes is an added bonus. I recommend liberal use of extra virgin olive oil when cooking and preparing meals.

References

1. American Heart Association (AHA). http://circ.ahajournals.org/content/123/4/e18.full.pdf. Accessed 27 May 2011.
2. Krauss RM, Deckelbaum RJ, Ernst N, Fisher E, Howard BV, Knopp RH, et al. Dietary guidelines for healthy American adults. A statement for health professionals from the Nutrition Committee, American Heart Association. Circulation. 1996;94(7):1795–800.
3. Anon. Mortality after 10 1/2 years for hypertensive participants in the Multiple Risk Factor Intervention Trial, "MRFIT". Circulation. 1990;82(5):1616–28.
4. Genest JJ, McNamara JR, Salem DN, Schaefer EJ. Prevalence of risk factors in men with premature coronary artery disease. Am J Cardiol. 1991;67(15):1185–9.

5. Dietary Guidelines for Americans Advisory Committee (DGAC) 2010. U.S. Department of Agriculture. Center for Nutrition Policy and Promotion. Dietary guidelines for Americans, 2010. http://www.cnpp.usda.gov/dietaryguidelines.htm. Accessed 1 Jan 2011.

6. Azadbakht L, Mirmiran P, Hedayati M, Esmaillzadeh A, Shiva N, Azizi F. Particle size of LDL is affected by the National Cholesterol Education Program (NCEP) step II diet in dyslipidaemic adolescents. Br J Nutr. 2007;98(1):134–9.

7. Berglund L, Lefevre M, Ginsberg HN, Kris-Etherton PM, Elmer PJ, Stewart PW, et al. DELTA Investigators. Comparison of monounsaturated fat with carbohydrates as a replacement for saturated fat in subjects with a high metabolic risk profile: studies in the fasting and postprandial states. Am J Clin Nutr. 2007;86(6):1611–20.

8. Chen SC, Judd JT, Kramer M, Meijer GW, Clevidence BA, Baer DJ. Phytosterol intake and dietary fat reduction are independent and additive in their ability to reduce plasma LDL cholesterol. Lipids. 2009;44(3):273–81.

9. Furtado JD, Campos H, Appel LJ, Miller ER, Laranjo N, Carey VJ, Sacks FM. Effect of protein, unsaturated fat, and carbohydrate intakes on plasma apolipoprotein B and VLDL and LDL containing apolipoprotein C-III: results from the OmniHeart Trial. Am J Clin Nutr. 2008;87(6):1623–36.

10. Galgani JE, Uauy RD, Aguirre CA, Díaz EO. Effect of the dietary fat quality on insulin sensitivity. Br J Nutr. 2008;100(3):471–9.

11. Jakobsen MU, O'Reilly EJ, Heitmann BL, Pereira MA, Bälter K, Fraser GE, et al. Major types of dietary fat and risk of coronary heart disease: a pooled analysis of 11 cohort studies. Am J Clin Nutr. 2009;89(5):1425–32.

12. Kralova Lesna I, Suchanek P, Kovar J, Stavek P, Poledne R. Replacement of dietary saturated FAs by PUFAs in diet and reverse cholesterol transport. J Lipid Res. 2008;49(11):2414–8.

13. Lichtenstein AH, Matthan NR, Jalbert SM, Resteghini NA, Schaefer EJ, Ausman LM. Novel soybean oils with different fatty acid profiles alter cardiovascular disease risk factors in moderately hyperlipidemic subjects. Am J Clin Nutr. 2006;84(3):497–504.

14. Lindström J, Ilanne-Parikka P, Peltonen M, Aunola S, Eriksson JG, Hemiö K, Finnish Diabetes Prevention Study Group, et al. Sustained reduction in the incidence of type 2 diabetes by lifestyle intervention: follow-up of the Finnish Diabetes Prevention Study. Lancet. 2006;368(9548):1673–9.

15. López S, Bermúdez B, Pacheco YM, Villar J, Abia R, Muriana FJ. Distinctive postprandial modulation of beta cell function and insulin sensitivity by dietary fats: monounsaturated compared with saturated fatty acids. Am J Clin Nutr. 2008;88(3):638–44.

16. Paniagua JA, de la Sacristana AG, Sánchez E, Romero I, Vidal-Puig A, Berral FJ, et al. A MUFA-rich diet improves posprandial glucose, lipid and GLP-1 responses in insulin-resistant subjects. J Am Coll Nutr. 2007;26(5):434–44.

17. Pérez-Jiménez F, López-Miranda J, Pinillos MD, Gómez P, Paz-Rojas E, Montilla P, et al. A Mediterranean and a high-carbohydrate diet improve glucose metabolism in healthy young persons. Diabetologia. 2001;44(11):2038–43.

18. Salmerón J, Hu FB, Manson JE, Stampfer MJ, Colditz GA, Rimm EB, Willett WC. Dietary fat intake and risk of type 2 diabetes in women. Am J Clin Nutr. 2001;73(6):1019–26.

19. Allman-Farinelli MA, Gomes K, Favaloro EJ, Petocz P. A diet rich in high-oleic-acid sunflower oil favorably alters low-density lipoprotein cholesterol, triglycerides, and factor VII coagulant activity. J Am Diet Assoc. 2005;105(7):1071–9.

20. Appel LJ, Sacks FM, Carey VJ, Obarzanek E, Swain JF, Miller 3rd ER, OmniHeart Collaborative Research Group, et al. Effects of protein, monounsaturated fat, and carbohydrate intake on blood pressure and serum lipids: results of the OmniHeart randomized trial. JAMA. 2005;294(19):2455–64.

21. Berglund L, Lefevre M, Ginsberg HN, Kris-Etherton PM, Elmer PJ, Stewart PW, et al. DELTA Investigators. Comparison of monounsaturated fat with carbohydrates as a replacement for saturated fat in subjects with a high metabolic risk profile: studies in the fasting and postprandial states. Am J Clin Nutr. 2007;86(6):1611–20.

22. Rasmussen BM, Vessby B, Uusitupa M, Berglund L, Pedersen E, Riccardi G, KANWU Study Group, et al. Effects of dietary saturated, monounsaturated, and n-3 fatty acids on blood pressure in healthy subjects. Am J Clin Nutr. 2006;83(2):221–6.
23. Tanasescu M, Cho E, Manson JE, Hu FB. Dietary fat and cholesterol and the risk of cardiovascular disease among women with type 2 diabetes. Am J Clin Nutr. 2004;79(6):999–1005.
24. Binkoski AE, Kris-Etherton PM, Wilson TA, Mountain ML, Nicolosi RJ. Balance of unsaturated fatty acids is important to a cholesterol-lowering diet: comparison of mid-oleic sunflower oil and olive oil on cardiovascular disease risk factors. J Am Diet Assoc. 2005;105(7): 1080–6.
25. Jakobsen MU, O'Reilly EJ, Heitmann BL, Pereira MA, Bälter K, Fraser GE, et al. Major types of dietary fat and risk of coronary heart disease: a pooled analysis of 11 cohort studies. Am J Clin Nutr. 2009;89(5):1425–32.
26. Mozaffarian D, Katan MB, Ascherio A, Stampfer MJ, Willett WC. Trans fatty acids and cardiovascular disease. N Engl J Med. 2006;354(15):1601–13.
27. Danaei G, Ding EL, Mozaffarian D, Taylor B, Rehm J, Murray CJ, Ezzati M. The preventable causes of death in the United States: comparative risk assessment of dietary, lifestyle, and metabolic risk factors. PLoS Med. 2009;6(4):e1000058.
28. St-Onge MP, Aban I, Bosarge A, Gower B, Hecker KD, Allison DB. Snack chips fried in corn oil alleviate cardiovascular disease risk factors when substituted for low-fat or high-fat snacks. Am J Clin Nutr. 2007;85(6):1503–10.
29. Zhao G, Etherton TD, Martin KR, West SG, Gillies PJ, Kris-Etherton PM. Dietary alpha-linolenic acid reduces inflammatory and lipid cardiovascular risk factors in hypercholesterolemic men and women. J Nutr. 2004;134(11):2991–7.
30. Burdge G. Alpha-linolenic acid metabolism in men and women: nutritional and biological implications. Curr Opin Clin Nutr Metab Care. 2004;7(2):137–44.
31. Institute of Medicine Fact Sheet, October 2006. http://www.iom.edu/~/media/Files/Report%20 Files/2006/Seafood-Choices-Balancing-Benefits-and-Risks/11762_SeafoodChoicesFact Sheet.pdf. Accessed 2 Dec 2011.
32. Monterey Bay Aquarium. http://www.montereybayaquarium.org/cr/cr_seafoodwatch/download.aspx. Accessed 27 May 2011.
33. Natural Resources Defense Council. http://www.nrdc.org/oceans/seafoodguide/. Accessed 27 May 2011.
34. Environmental Defense Fund. www.edf.org/seafoodhealth. Accessed 27 May 2011.
35. O'Keefe Jr JH, Cordain L, Harris WH, Moe RM, Vogel R. Optimal low-density lipoprotein is 50 to 70 mg/dl: lower is better and physiologically normal. J Am Coll Cardiol. 2004;43(11):2142–6.
36. Harman NL, Leeds AR, Griffin BA. Increased dietary cholesterol does not increase plasma low density lipoprotein when accompanied by an energy-restricted diet and weight loss. Eur J Nutr. 2008;47(6):287–93.
37. Greene CM, Zern TL, Wood RJ, Shrestha S, Aggarwal D, Sharman MJ, et al. Maintenance of the LDL cholesterol:HDL cholesterol ratio in an elderly population given a dietary cholesterol challenge. J Nutr. 2005;135(12):2793–8.
38. Goodrow EF, Wilson TA, Houde SC, Vishwanathan R, Scollin PA, Handelman G, Nicolosi RJ. Consumption of one egg per day increases serum lutein and zeaxanthin concentrations in older adults without altering serum lipid and lipoprotein cholesterol concentrations. J Nutr. 2006;136(10):2519–24.
39. Weggemans RM, Zock PL, Katan MB. Dietary cholesterol from eggs increases the ratio of total cholesterol to high-density lipoprotein cholesterol in humans: a meta-analysis. Am J Clin Nutr. 2001;73(5):885–91.
40. Nakamura Y, Iso H, Kita Y, Ueshima H, Okada K, Konishi M, et al. Egg consumption, serum total cholesterol concentrations and coronary heart disease incidence: Japan Public Health Center-based prospective study. Br J Nutr. 2006;96(5):921–8.
41. Qureshi AI, Suri FK, Ahmed S, Nasar A, Divani AA, Kirmani JF. Regular egg consumption does not increase the risk of stroke and cardiovascular diseases. Med Sci Monit. 2007;13(1):CR1–8.

42. Hu FB, Stampfer MJ, Rimm EB, Manson JE, Ascherio A, Colditz GA, et al. A prospective study of egg consumption and risk of cardiovascular disease in men and women. JAMA. 1999;281(15):1387–94.
43. Hu FB, Stampfer MJ, Manson JE, Rimm EB, Wolk A, Colditz GA, et al. Dietary intake of alpha-linolenic acid and risk of fatal ischemic heart disease among women. Am J Clin Nutr. 1999;69(5):890–7.
44. Kritchevsky SB, Kritchevsky D. Egg consumption and coronary heart disease: an epidemiologic overview. J Am Coll Nutr. 2000;19(5 Suppl):549S–55S.
45. Clarke R, Frost C, Collins R, Appleby P, Peto R. Dietary lipids and blood cholesterol: quantitative meta-analysis of metabolic ward studies. BMJ. 1997;314(7074):112–7.
46. Perez-Jimenez F, de Alvarez Cienfuegos G, Badimon L, Barja G, Battino M, Blanco A, et al. International conference on the healthy effect of virgin olive oil. Eur J Clin Invest. 2005;35(7):421–4.
47. Huang CL, Sumpio BE. Olive oil, the Mediterranean diet, and cardiovascular health. J Am Coll Surg. 2008;207(3):407–16.
48. USDA Food Bank. www.nal.usda.gov/fnic/foodcomp/data/food. Accessed 27 May 2011.

Chapter 12
Carbohydrates

Keywords Mediterranean diet • Carbohydrates • Sugar • Starch • Fiber
• Glycemic index

Carbohydrates provide four calories of energy per gram, and they are the major source of energy in the human diet. They exist as sugars, starches, and fibers in a diverse group of foods. Mediterranean diet studies address the fact that there is a distinction between biological actions of carbohydrates by counting some sources favorably and others unfavorably in calculating a MedDiet-adherence score (AS). Carbohydrate-rich whole foods such as fruits, vegetables, legumes, and whole grains contribute favorably to a MedDiet-AS whereas processed and refined carbohydrate-containing foods such as sugar or high-fructose corn syrup sweetened beverages, refined flours and sugars in dessert foods, and white rice contribute unfavorably to a MedDiet-AS.

I usually explain the nomenclature of carbohydrates before discussing them in depth with patients since the different terms will frequently be encountered both in the popular and scientific press. The nomenclature for carbohydrates begins by dividing them into the two major subgroups: complex and simple. Simple carbohydrates contain the monosaccharide and disaccharide groups (Table 12.1 and Fig. 12.1). Monosaccharides are comprised of a single sugar unit and are the simplest carbohydrates. The three important monosaccharides in human nutrition are glucose, fructose, and galactose. Monosaccharides cannot be broken into simpler sugar units, and they form the building blocks for all other carbohydrates. Disaccharides are comprised of two monosaccharides bonded together. The three naturally occurring disaccharides in human nutrition are sucrose, lactose, and maltose. These contain glucose bonded to fructose, glucose bonded to galactose, and glucose bonded to glucose, respectively. High-fructose corn syrup is a manmade disaccharide created by the hydrolysis of corn and contains fructose bonded to fructose.

E. Zacharias, *The Mediterranean Diet: A Clinician's Guide for Patient Care*,
DOI 10.1007/978-1-4614-3326-2_12, © Springer Science+Business Media, LLC 2012

Table 12.1 Simple carbohydrates

Simple carbohydrates: monosaccharides and disaccharides	
Monosaccharides: single sugar units	
Glucose	
Fructose	
Galactose	
Disaccharides: two monosaccharides bonded together	
	Bonded
Sucrose	Glucose–fructose
Lactose	Glucose–galactose
Maltose	Glucose–glucose
High fructose corn syrup	Fructose–fructose

The nomenclature of complex carbohydrates, those with three or more monosaccharides bonded together, is simplified by organizing them into two major groups: the oligosaccharides and polysaccharides (Table 12.2 and Fig. 12.1). The oligosaccharides contain three to ten monosaccharides bonded together and the polysaccharides contain greater that ten monosaccharides bonded together. There are three main dietary oligosaccharides: raffinose made of sucrose bonded to galactose, stachyose made of raffinose bonded to galactose, and verbacose made of stachyose bonded to galactose.

Polysaccharides are divided into three major categories: starches, glycogen, and dietary fibers. Starches are the principle storage form of carbohydrate in plants and are found in a variety of foods including vegetables, beans, and grains. They are polymers of amylose and amylopectin, both of which are polymers of glucose, and they are generally digestible by humans. Glycogen is also a polymer of glucose, and it is the only polysaccharide of animal origin where it serves as the main storage form of carbohydrate. Glycogen is readily metabolized to its glucose building blocks to meet energy demands of the body. The final category of polysaccharides, the dietary fibers, contains myriad different compounds all of which are complex polymers of monosaccharides, and they are only partially digestible by humans. Fibers are often further categorized as soluble or insoluble. The soluble fibers include pectin, gums, beta-glucans, and some hemicelluloses, and the insoluble fibers include lignin, cellulose, and some hemicelluloses.

Importance of Fibers: Intrinsic and a Marker for Whole Foods

Dietary fibers are important nutrients contained within many of the whole food carbohydrate sources that contribute favorably to calculating a MedDiet-AS. When carbohydrate sources such as whole grains are processed and refined, the fibers containing components are partially or completely removed (Fig. 12.2).

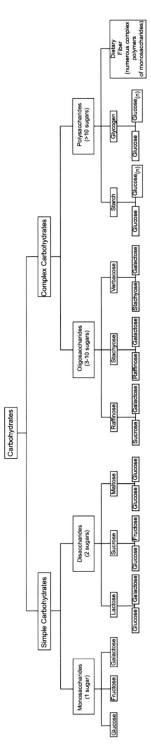

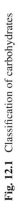

Fig. 12.1 Classification of carbohydrates

Table 12.2 Complex carbohydrates

Complex carbohydrates: oligosaccharides and polysaccharides	
Oligosaccharides: 3–10 monosaccharides bonded together	
	Bonded
Raffinose	Sucrose (glucose–fructose)–galactose
Stachyose	Sucrose (glucose–fructose)–(galactose)$_2$
Verbacose	Sucrose (glucose–fructose)–(galactose)$_3$
Polysaccharides: greater than 10 monosaccharides bonded together	
Starches	Glucose–(glucose)$_n$
Glycogen	Glucose–(glucose)$_n$
Dietary fibers	Myriad polymers of monosaccharides

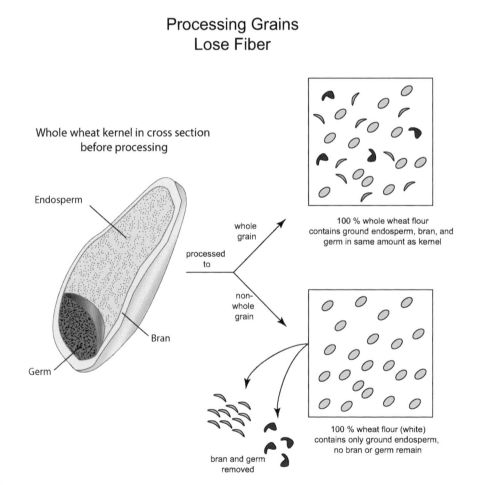

Fig. 12.2 Processing causes grains to lose fiber

Prior to refining, whole grains contain all of a grain's edible parts, the bran, germ, and endosperm with all of their intrinsic fibers and biologically active phytochemicals [1].

Dietary fibers can have several beneficial effects on health. The fibers present in whole food sources act in the stomach to delay gastric emptying time and to promote the sensation of satiety. This may result in a reduction in total caloric consumption. For example, consuming a fiber-rich whole apple has been demonstrated to reduce subsequent energy consumption significantly more than an equal number of calories from very low-fiber apple juice [2]. Slowed gastric emptying caused by fiber-rich foods also prolongs intestinal absorption of digested sugars so the body experiences a more gradual rise and fall in postprandial blood glucose levels. A gradual rise in blood glucose reduces hyperinsulinemia and the subsequent postprandial hyperadrenergic counter-regulatory response that occurs after rapid spikes in glucose levels [3]. Fibers also bind intestinal bile acids and intestinal lipids, which helps to reduce serum lipid levels [3]. The water-holding property of fibers serves to increase fecal volume so that ease and volume of defecation is improved and constipation is reduced. This may also reduce development of diverticulosis. Intestinal bacteria partially metabolize dietary fibers, and this may promote a healthy colonic microenvironment favorable to normal colonic mucosal cells and reduce the risk of their cancerous transformation [3].

The high fiber categories in a MedDiet—such as vegetables, fruits, whole grains, and legumes—are important to health because, as noted previously, diets with adequate fiber have been linked to reduced risk of cardiovascular disease (CVD), diabetes, colon cancer, and obesity [3–8]. Whether these benefits are from the fibers per se or from the total benefits of the overall nutrient profiles of whole foods containing the fibers such as fruits, vegetables, whole grains, and legumes is impossible to distinguish. Most likely, both are important. When reviewing information regarding their important biological effects, fibers may be thought of as markers for consumption of whole fruits, vegetables, legumes, and grains.

Reporting in the lay press on the benefits or lack of benefits shown in clinical trials of fiber consumption may lead to confusion in patients. The distinction I make with patients is that the fibers contained in a MedDiet are obtained from whole, plant-source foods, and their favorable health impacts occur in the context of an entire dietary pattern, not when taken as an isolated supplemental nutrient. If the source of the fibers in a clinical trial was from a fiber supplement as opposed to whole foods, then participants would experience most of the mechanical benefits of fibers, but miss out on the potential benefits obtained from the hundreds of biologically active phytochemicals that come with the fibers in whole foods. Americans are doing a poor job of consuming adequate fiber. A recent report showed that, except for in women aged 50 years or greater, fewer than 5% of Americans consume the recommended amount of fiber [9]. As part of a complete, well-balanced dietary approach, increased consumption of plant-based foods rich in fiber, such as whole grains, vegetables, fruits, beans, and nuts (Table 12.3), contributes to the health-promoting effects observed with a MedDiet.

Table 12.3 Fiber content of common foods

Food	Gram of fiber/100 g
Pinto beans	15.5
Kidney beans	15.2
Black beans	15.2
Almonds	12.2
Pecans	9.6
Walnuts	6.7
Bread, whole wheat	6
Cashews	3.3
Pear	3.1
Quinoa	2.8
Banana	2.6
Peas	2.6
Potato, with skin	2.5
Apple	2.4
Orange	2.4
Blueberries	2.4
Bread, white	2.3
Flour, whole wheat	2.3
Asparagus	2.1
Amaranth	2.1
Strawberries	2
Oatmeal	1.9
Rice, brown	1.8
Broccoli	1.5
Peach	1.5
Mushrooms	1.3
Corn	1
Grapes	0.9
Rice, white	0.3
Flour, white	0.3

Glycemic Index

The glycemic index (GI) is a term that I have been asked about with increasing frequency when discussing carbohydrates with patients. Glycemic index is defined as the amount that a food, consumed alone and in a fasting state, will raise blood glucose over a 2-h period of time relative to a reference carbohydrate. The reference carbohydrate, by definition given a GI value of 100, is usually white bread. Individual carbohydrate sources have an intrinsic GI value, but the actual effect a food has on blood glucose depends on many variables. If a food was consumed in isolation as when its GI is calculated, then its GI would be significantly higher than its effective GI when consumed as part of a meal along with other fats, proteins, and carbohydrates. This is because the presence of other foods in the stomach and intestines affects gastric emptying rate and intestinal absorption rates. For example,

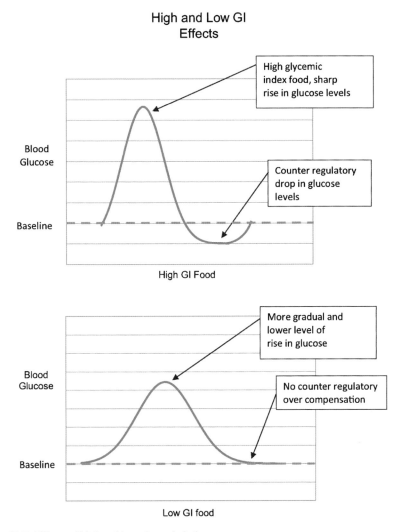

Fig. 12.3 Effects of high and low glycemic index

olive oil on bread will lower the bread's GI by delaying gastric emptying. The same effect would occur with bread's effective GI as part of a peanut butter or turkey sandwich. Thus, although carbohydrate sources have an intrinsic GI, their effective GI depends on the context in which they are consumed (Fig. 12.3).

The health importance of selecting foods with a certain GI has yet to be fully described, but it is reasonable to follow a MedDiet that avoids large amounts of simple and refined carbohydrates, with their high GIs, if one is interested in reducing dietary GI. There are several theoretical reasons lowering GI may be of benefit. Except during periods of vigorous physical exertion, the spike in blood glucose

Table 12.4 Reducing the glycemic index (GI)

How to reduce glycemic index of diet
Avoid foods with added sugars
Choose fruits for sweets, as fiber lowers GI
Choose whole grains and whole grain flours over processed and refined flours
If consuming foods with relatively high GI, then add healthy fat source and/or healthy protein source to lower effective GI

caused by overconsumption of high GI foods can lead to a hyperinsulinemic response. This exaggerated rise in insulin levels causes a postprandial hyperadrenergic, counter-regulatory response and may result in unpleasant symptoms including tachycardia, tremor, sweating, weakness, and difficulty with concentrating. These counter-regulatory hormone surges also promote the release of free fatty acids from adipose tissue that then increase serum triglyceride and very low-density lipoprotein (VLDL) levels [10]. This cascade of events is one of the reasons simple carbohydrates can elevate serum lipid levels even though they contain no fat themselves. The effect of high GI foods also has theoretically, but as yet unproven, adverse effects on risk for CVD, T2D, and cancer. Based upon their review of 55 studies examining the relationship between GI and disease, the DGAC 2010 has concluded that there currently is insufficient evidence to suggest a direct relationship between a food's GI and risk for CVD, T2D, or cancer [3]. Additionally, although some short-term trials of under 8 weeks duration have shown benefit in weight loss with low GI diets [11, 12], numerous longer term trials, 16 weeks or greater, have shown no difference between high and low glycemic index diets in effects on weight [13–22]. See Chap. 9 for more information on the effects macronutrient balance has on weight control. While the topic of GI is undergoing further research, it is prudent to reduce consumption of foods with a high GI, particularly in isolation, with well-balanced, whole food sources as in a MedDiet (Table 12.4).

Reduced or low-carbohydrate diets have enjoyed intermittent popularity over the years for their purported weight loss and health benefits, and health care providers should be prepared to address them when discussing carbohydrate sources in a MedDiet with patients. There are favorable health effects with restricting consumption of certain types of carbohydrates—specifically the simple, processed, and refined sugars and white flours—but it is detrimental to health to restrict carbohydrates from vegetables, fruits, whole grains, nuts, or legumes. A common observation from patients is that when they begin carbohydrate restriction they experience weight loss. This is indeed often the case as simple sugars are often the main source of caloric overconsumption. However, the rapid loss of large amounts of weight that patients report, out of proportion to the amount of caloric reduction, is caused by excretion of water that is normally bound to stored glycogen and not loss of large amounts of fat. The actual reduction in adiposity that occurs with carbohydrate restriction reflects caloric reduction while any additional weight loss is simply water weight that will re-equilibrate over time. Carbohydrate-restricting diets have not been shown to be superior to other dietary strategies for long-term weight loss [3, 23, 24]. See Chap. 9 for an in-depth discussion of macronutrient content of diet and effects on body weight.

From both a disease prevention and weight loss standpoint, Americans do indeed obtain too many their calories from processed and refined carbohydrate sources, the so-called "bad carbohydrates," so restricting these makes sense in any diet. If other calories are not consumed in the place of these sugars, then, by definition patients restricting carbohydrates will experience the weight benefits that come from a negative energy balance. However, analogous to a dietary strategy of avoiding all fats, the dietary strategy of avoiding all carbohydrates misses the key point that there are significant differences among types and sources of carbohydrates. Individuals should consume health-promoting whole food carbohydrate sources, rich in dietary fibers and biologically active micronutrients, and avoid the "bad carbohydrates," particularly simple sugars including high fructose corn syrup and refined grains, which can have a deleterious effect on health and weight control.

Studies/Trials

Whole grains, fruits, legumes, and vegetables are carbohydrate sources in a MedDiet of common interest, and studies showing their health benefits are briefly summarized here.

Numerous published studies have shown an association between whole grain intake and reduced CVD [3, 25–29], reduced type 2 diabetes (T2D) [30–32], and reduced body weight [33–38]. Increased consumption of fruits and vegetables is associated with reduced risk for CVD, and there may be a dose–response effect with greater reduction in CVD seen at higher consumption levels [39–44]. In an assessment of dietary risk factors, low consumption of fruits and vegetables was determined to account for 55,000 preventable deaths each year [45]. Numerous recent studies have also shown reduction in weight with increased consumption of fruits and vegetables; however, it remains to be proven that these benefits are sustainable for a long period of time [46–56]. Several studies have shown an inverse association between increased fruits, consumption of vegetables, or both on risk for T2D [57–59]. A comprehensive review of relevant literature and subsequent report of the World Cancer Research Fund and the American Institute for Cancer Research concluded that nonstarchy vegetables alone or in combination with fruits were associated with reduced cancer risk and possibly had a dose–response effect [60]. Unfortunately, in the United States, fewer than 20% of men and 29% of women consume five servings or more of combined total of fruits and vegetables per day [61] (Fig. 12.4).

In conclusion, the carbohydrate macronutrient class is the body's chief source of energy and is critical to life. A MedDiet encourages the preponderance of carbohydrates consumed come from whole food source vegetables, legumes, fruits, and whole grains.

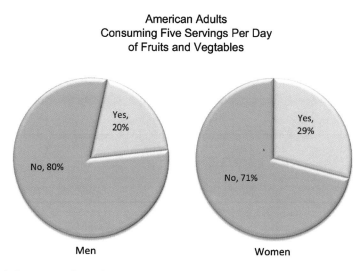

**American Adults
Consuming Five Servings Per Day
of Fruits and Vegtables**

Men   Women

Fig. 12.4 Percentage of American adults consuming five or more servings of fruits and vegetables per day

References

1. Jacobs Jr DR, Steffen LM. Nutrients, foods, and dietary patterns as exposures in research: a framework for food synergy. Am J Clin Nutr. 2003;78(3 Suppl):508S–13.
2. Flood-Obbagy JE, Rolls BJ. The effect of fruit in different forms on energy intake and satiety at a meal. Appetite. 2009;52(2):416–22.
3. Dietary Guidelines for Americans Advisory Committee (DGAC) 2010. U.S. Department of Agriculture. Center for Nutrition Policy and Promotion. Dietary guidelines for Americans, 2010. http://www.cnpp.usda.gov/dietaryguidelines.htm. Accessed 1 Jan 2011.
4. Slavin JL. Position of the American Dietetic Association: health implications of dietary fiber. J Am Diet Assoc. 2008;108(10):1716–31.
5. Du H, van der A DL, Boshuizen HC, Forouhi NG, Wareham NJ, Halkjaer J, et al. Dietary fiber and subsequent changes in body weight and waist circumference in European men and women. Am J Clin Nutr. 2010;91(2):329–36.
6. Tucker LA, Thomas KS. Increasing total fiber intake reduces risk of weight and fat gains in women. J Nutr. 2009;139(3):576–81.
7. Davis JN, Alexander KE, Ventura EE, Toledo-Corral CM, Goran MI. Inverse relation between dietary fiber intake and visceral adiposity in overweight Latino youth. Am J Clin Nutr. 2009;90(5):1160–6.
8. Hopping BN, Erber E, Grandinetti A, Verheus M, Kolonel LN, Maskarinec G. Dietary fiber, magnesium, and glycemic load alter risk of type 2 diabetes in a multiethnic cohort in Hawaii. J Nutr. 2010;140(1):68–74.
9. Marriott BP, Olsho L, Hadden L, Connor P. Intake of added sugars and selected nutrients in the United States, National Health and Nutrition Examination Survey (NHANES) 2003–2006. Crit Rev Food Sci Nutr. 2010;50:228–58.
10. Ludwig DS. The glycemic index: physiological mechanisms relating to obesity, diabetes, and cardiovascular disease. JAMA. 2002;287(18):2414–23.
11. Abete I, Parra D, Crujeiras AB, Goyenechea E, Martinez JA. Specific insulin sensitivity and leptin responses to a nutritional treatment of obesity via a combination of energy restriction and fatty fish intake. J Hum Nutr Diet. 2008;21(6):591–600.

12. de Rougemont A, Normand S, Nazare JA, Skilton MR, Sothier M, Vinoy S, Laville M. Beneficial effects of a 5-week low-glycaemic index regimen on weight control and cardiovascular risk factors in overweight non-diabetic subjects. Br J Nutr. 2007;98(6):1288–98.

13. Philippou E, Neary NM, Chaudhri O, Brynes AE, Dornhorst A, Leeds AR, Hickson M, Frost GS. The effect of dietary glycemic index on weight maintenance in overweight subjects: a pilot study. Obesity (Silver Spring). 2009;17(2):396–401.

14. Pittas AG, Roberts SB, Das SK, Gilhooly CH, Saltzman E, Golden J, Stark PC, Greenberg AS. The effects of the dietary glycemic load on type 2 diabetes risk factors during weight loss. Obesity (Silver Spring). 2006;14(12):2200–9.

15. Raatz SK, Torkelson CJ, Redmon JB, Reck KP, Kwong CA, Swanson JE, Liu C, Thomas W, Bantle JP. Reduced glycemic index and glycemic load diets do not increase the effects of energy restriction on weight loss and insulin sensitivity in obese men and women. J Nutr. 2005;135(10):2387–91.

16. Sichieri R, Moura AS, Genelhu V, Hu F, Willett WC. An 18-mo randomized trial of a low-glycemic-index diet and weight change in Brazilian women. Am J Clin Nutr. 2007;86(3):707–13.

17. Sloth B, Krog-Mikkelsen I, Flint A, Tetens I, Björck I, Vinoy S, Elmståhl H, Astrup A, Lang V, Raben A. No difference in body weight decrease between a low-glycemic-index and a high-glycemic-index diet but reduced LDL cholesterol after 10-wk ad libitum intake of the low-glycemic-index diet. Am J Clin Nutr. 2004;80(2):337–47.

18. Ebbeling CB, Leidig MM, Feldman HA, Lovesky MM, Ludwig DS. Effects of a low-glycemic load vs low-fat diet in obese young adults: a randomized trial. JAMA. 2007;297(19):2092–102; Erratum in: JAMA. 2007;298(6):627.

19. Maki KC, Rains TM, Kaden VN, Raneri KR, Davidson MH. Effects of a reduced-glycemic-load diet on body weight, body composition, and cardiovascular disease risk markers in overweight and obese adults. Am J Clin Nutr. 2007;85(3):724–34.

20. Pereira MA, Swain J, Goldfine AB, Rifai N, Ludwig DS. Effects of a low-glycemic load diet on resting energy expenditure and heart disease risk factors during weight loss. JAMA. 2004;292(20):2482–90.

21. Pal S, Lim S, Egger G. The effect of a low glycaemic index breakfast on blood glucose, insulin, lipid profiles, blood pressure, body weight, body composition and satiety in obese and overweight individuals: a pilot study. J Am Coll Nutr. 2008;27(3):387–93.

22. McMillan-Price J, Petocz P, Atkinson F, O'neill K, Samman S, Steinbeck K, Caterson I, Brand-Miller J. Comparison of 4 diets of varying glycemic load on weight loss and cardiovascular risk reduction in overweight and obese young adults: a randomized controlled trial. Arch Intern Med. 2006;166(14):1466–75.

23. Centers for Disease Control and Prevention. National Health and Nutrition Examination Survey, NHANES, 2000–2005. www.cdc.gov/nchs/nhanes. Accessed 27 May 2011.

24. Miller DS, Judd PA. The metabolisable energy value of foods. J Sci Food Agric. 1984;35:111–6.

25. Kelly SA, Summerbell CD, Brynes A, Whittaker V, Frost G. Wholegrain cereals for coronary heart disease. Cochrane Database Syst Rev. 2007;(2):CD005051.

26. Mellen PB, Walsh TF, Herrington DM. Whole grain intake and cardiovascular disease: a meta-analysis. Nutr Metab Cardiovasc Dis. 2008;18(4):283–90.

27. Flint AJ, Hu FB, Glynn RJ, Jensen MK, Franz M, Sampson L, Rimm EB. Whole grains and incident hypertension in men. Am J Clin Nutr. 2009;90(3):493–8.

28. Djoussé L, Gaziano JM. Breakfast cereals and risk of heart failure in the physicians' health study I. Arch Intern Med. 2007;167(19):2080–5.

29. Nettleton JA, Steffen LM, Loehr LR, Rosamond WD, Folsom AR. Incident heart failure is associated with lower whole-grain intake and greater high-fat dairy and egg intake in the Atherosclerosis Risk in Communities (ARIC) study. J Am Diet Assoc. 2008; 108(11):1881–7.

30. de Munter JS, Hu FB, Spiegelman D, Franz M, van Dam RM. Whole grain, bran, and germ intake and risk of type 2 diabetes: a prospective cohort study and systematic review. PLoS Med. 2007;4(8):e261.

31. Priebe MG, van Binsbergen JJ, de Vos R, Vonk RJ. Whole grain foods for the prevention of type 2 diabetes mellitus. Cochrane Database Syst Rev. 2008;(1):CD006061.
32. Kochar J, Djoussé L, Gaziano JM. Breakfast cereals and risk of type 2 diabetes in the Physicians' Health Study I. Obesity (Silver Spring). 2007;15(12):3039–44.
33. Harland JI, Garton LE. Whole-grain intake as a marker of healthy body weight and adiposity. Whole-grain intake as a marker of healthy body weight and adiposity. Public Health Nutr. 2008;11(6):554–63.
34. Williams PG, Grafenauer SJ, O'Shea JE. Cereal grains, legumes, and weight management: a comprehensive review of the scientific evidence. Nutr Rev. 2008;66(4):171–82.
35. Behall KM, Scholfield DJ, Hallfrisch J. Whole-grain diets reduce blood pressure in mildly hypercholesterolemic men and women. J Am Diet Assoc. 2006;106(9):1445–9.
36. Lutsey PL, Jacobs Jr DR, Kori S, Mayer-Davis E, Shea S, Steffen LM, Szklo M, Tracy R. Whole grain intake and its cross-sectional association with obesity, insulin resistance, inflammation, diabetes and subclinical CVD: the MESA Study. Br J Nutr. 2007; 98(2):397–405.
37. McKeown NM, Yoshida M, Shea MK, Jacques PF, Lichtenstein AH, Rogers G, Booth SL, Saltzman E. Whole-grain intake and cereal fiber are associated with lower abdominal adiposity in older adults. J Nutr. 2009;139(10):1950–5.
38. van de Vijver LP, van den Bosch LM, van den Brandt PA, Goldbohm RA. Whole-grain consumption, dietary fibre intake and body mass index in the Netherlands cohort study. Eur J Clin Nutr. 2009;63(1):31–8.
39. Dauchet L, Amouyel P, Dallongeville J. Fruit and vegetable consumption and risk of stroke: a meta-analysis of cohort studies. Neurology. 2005;65(8):1193–7.
40. Dauchet L, Amouyel P, Hercberg S, Dallongeville J. Fruit and vegetable consumption and risk of coronary heart disease: a meta-analysis of cohort studies. J Nutr. 2006;136(10):2588–93.
41. Genkinger JM, Platz EA, Hoffman SC, Comstock GW, Helzlsouer KJ. Fruit, vegetable, and antioxidant intake and all-cause, cancer, and cardiovascular disease mortality in a community-dwelling population in Washington County, Maryland. Am J Epidemiol. 2004;160(12):1223–33.
42. Hung HC, Joshipura KJ, Jiang R, Hu FB, Hunter D, Smith-Warner SA, Colditz GA, Rosner B, Spiegelman D, Willett WC. Fruit and vegetable intake and risk of major chronic disease. J Natl Cancer Inst. 2004;96(21):1577–84.
43. Joshipura KJ, Hung HC, Li TY, Hu FB, Rimm EB, Stampfer MJ, Colditz G, Willett WC. Intakes of fruits, vegetables and carbohydrate and the risk of CVD. Public Health Nutr. 2009;12(1):115–21.
44. He FJ, Nowson CA, Lucas M, MacGregor GA. Increased consumption of fruit and vegetables is related to a reduced risk of coronary heart disease: meta-analysis of cohort studies. J Hum Hypertens. 2007;21(9):717–28.
45. Danaei G, Ding EL, Mozaffarian D, Taylor B, Rehm J, Murray CJ, Ezzati M. The preventable causes of death in the United States: comparative risk assessment of dietary, lifestyle, and metabolic risk factors. PLoS Med. 2009;6(4):e1000058.
46. Bes-Rastrollo M, Martínez-González MA, Sánchez-Villegas A, de la Fuente Arrillaga C, Martínez JA. Association of fiber intake and fruit/vegetable consumption with weight gain in a Mediterranean population. Nutrition. 2006;22(5):504–11.
47. Buijsse B, Feskens EJ, Schulze MB, Forouhi NG, Wareham NJ, Sharp S, Palli D, Tognon G, Halkjaer J, Tjønneland A, Jakobsen MU, Overvad K, van der A DL A, Du H, Sørensen TI, Boeing H. Fruit and vegetable intakes and subsequent changes in body weight in European populations: results from the project on diet, obesity, and genes (DiOGenes). Am J Clin Nutr. 2009;90(1):202–9.
48. Davis JN, Hodges VA, Gillham MB. Normal-weight adults consume more fiber and fruit than their age- and height-matched overweight/obese counterparts. J Am Diet Assoc. 2006; 106(6):833–40.
49. Fujioka K, Greenway F, Sheard J, Ying Y. The effects of grapefruit on weight and insulin resistance: relationship to the metabolic syndrome. J Med Food. 2006;9(1):49–54.

50. Goss J, Grubbs L. Comparative analysis of body mass index, consumption of fruits and vege-tables, smoking, and physical activity among Florida residents. J Community Health Nurs. 2005;22(1):37–46.
51. He K, Hu FB, Colditz GA, Manson JE, Willett WC, Liu S. Changes in intake of fruits and vegetables in relation to risk of obesity and weight gain among middle-aged women. Int J Obes Relat Metab Disord. 2004;28(12):1569–74.
52. Ortega RM, Rodríguez-Rodríguez E, Aparicio A, Marín-Arias LI, López-Sobaler AM. Responses to two weight-loss programs based on approximating the diet to the ideal: differ-ences associated with increased cereal or vegetable consumption. Int J Vitam Nutr Res. 2006;76(6):367–76.
53. Radhika G, Sudha V, Mohan Sathya R, Ganesan A, Mohan V. Association of fruit and vegeta-ble intake with cardiovascular risk factors in urban south Indians. Br J Nutr. 2008;99(2):398–405.
54. Tanumihardjo SA, Valentine AR, Zhang Z, Whigham LD, Lai HJ, Atkinson RL. Strategies to increase vegetable or reduce energy and fat intake induce weight loss in adults. Exp Biol Med (Maywood). 2009;234(5):542–52.
55. Vioque J, Weinbrenner T, Castelló A, Asensio L, Garcia de la Hera M. Intake of fruits and vegetables in relation to 10-year weight gain among Spanish adults. Obesity (Silver Spring). 2008;16(3):664–70.
56. Xu F, Yin XM, Tong SL. Association between excess bodyweight and intake of red meat and vegetables among urban and rural adult Chinese in Nanjing, China. Asia Pac J Public Health. 2007;19(3):3–9.
57. Liu S, Serdula M, Janket SJ, Cook NR, Sesso HD, Willett WC, Manson JE, Buring JE. A prospective study of fruit and vegetable intake and the risk of type 2 diabetes in women. Diabetes Care. 2004;27(12):2993–6.
58. Villegas R, Shu XO, Gao YT, Yang G, Elasy T, Li H, Zheng W. Vegetable but not fruit con-sumption reduces the risk of type 2 diabetes in Chinese women. J Nutr. 2008;138(3):574–80.
59. Bazzano LA, Li TY, Joshipura KJ, Hu FB. Intake of fruit, vegetables, and fruit juices and risk of diabetes in women. Diabetes Care. 2008;31(7):1311–7.
60. World Cancer Research Fund and the American Institute for Cancer Research. Food, nutrition, physical activity, and the prevention of cancer: a global perspective; 2007. http://www.dietand-cancerreport.org/. Accessed 27 May 2011.
61. Blanck HM, Gillespie C, Kimmons JE, Seymour JD, Serdula MK. Trends in fruit and vegetable consumption among U.S. men and women, 1994-2005. Prev Chronic Dis. 2008;5(2):A35.

Chapter 13
Proteins

Keywords Mediterranean diet • Amino acids • Protein synthesis • Peptide bonds • Polypeptides

The protein macronutrient class in a Mediterranean diet is supplied from diverse food sources—both plant and animal in origin. Dietary proteins may be thought of as the means by which adequate amino acids are supplied to meet the body's requirements for synthesis and repair of its protein-containing components. When calculating a Mediterranean diet adherence score, the high-intake, protein-rich categories include fish, lean poultry, fat free dairy, egg whites, legumes, nuts and seeds, and soy products. The low-intake, protein-rich categories include red meats, processed meat products, whole fat dairy, and egg yolks. A MedDiet, although not traditionally vegetarian, provides ample daily protein from multiple, nonanimal-flesh sources and is compatible with vegetarianism if a patient desires.

The most common question I get when advising a patient to significantly reduce his or her meat and meat product intake for health purposes is "… but where do I get my protein?" These patients are expressing the common concern that the desirable dietary change of reducing or eliminating meat and meat products might cause an inability to meet their body's daily protein requirements. A deeper understanding of proteins and protein sources outlined in this chapter will clarify this issue. As will be explained, it is nearly impossible with a balanced diet such as a MedDiet, with or without animal flesh foods, to consume less than adequate protein amounts. However, it can be challenging to explain this point in a concise fashion. This section of the book will give providers the basic information necessary to share with patients the science of protein requirements and metabolism and sources of dietary protein.

E. Zacharias, *The Mediterranean Diet: A Clinician's Guide for Patient Care,*
DOI 10.1007/978-1-4614-3326-2_13, © Springer Science+Business Media, LLC 2012

Nomenclature

A discussion of amino acids and protein synthesis lays the groundwork for explaining more complex concepts. Proteins are comprised of amino acids, and a unique side chain group differentiates the 20 amino acids from each other (Fig. 13.1).

In the process of forming a protein, amino acids are first linked together by peptide bonds creating long chains called polypeptides (Fig. 13.2).

Polypeptides then fold into complex conformations, may have additional functional groups attached to them, and ultimately take the form of a specific protein (Fig. 13.3).

Patients frequently encounter the terms essential (indispensable) amino acids, nonessential (dispensable) amino acids, limiting amino acids, complete proteins, incomplete proteins, and complementary proteins when reading dietary articles and books. My experience is that a lack of understanding of these terms often causes patients to be reluctant to reduce intake of meats and meat products. After going through the exercise of learning what these terms mean, patients tend to have more confidence that there is no risk of inadequate protein consumption in nearly any balanced diet. To understand these terms, a basic comprehension of protein synthesis is necessary (Fig. 13.4 graphically represents protein synthesis and may be used as a visual reference when reading the following description).

When a protein's synthesis is required, a process called DNA transcription is initiated in the cell's nucleus. This results in production of a strand of nucleic acids called messenger RNA (mRNA) using the DNA as a template. Next, the mRNA leaves the cell's nucleus and enters the cytoplasm where its nucleic acids are read three-at-a-time, and in sequence, by a ribosome. Each three nucleic acid group read simultaneously is referred to as a codon, or triplet code, and is specific for one amino acid. When the codon is read, its matching anticodon on transfer RNA (tRNA) takes an amino acid that corresponds to the codon from the body's "amino acid pool" and delivers it to the mRNA and ribosome. Then, the next codon is read, and that codon's corresponding tRNA delivers the specific amino acid coded for from the amino acid pool. The two amino acids are then bonded together by a peptide bond. This process continues with the third delivered amino acid bonding to the second and so on until all of the amino acids have been delivered in sequence and

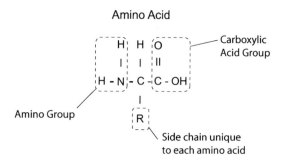

Fig. 13.1 Amino acid

Peptide and Polypeptide

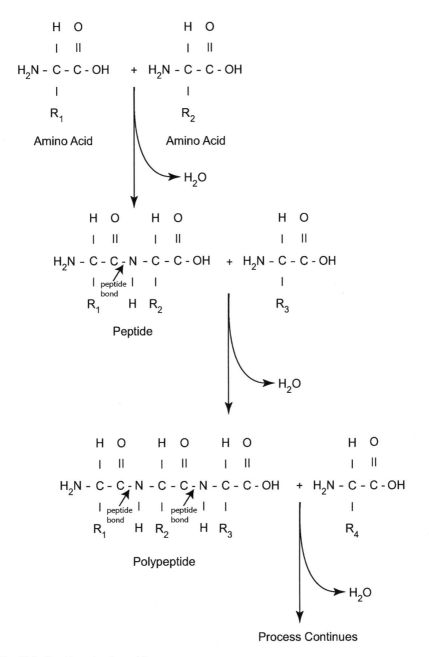

Fig. 13.2 Peptide and polypeptide

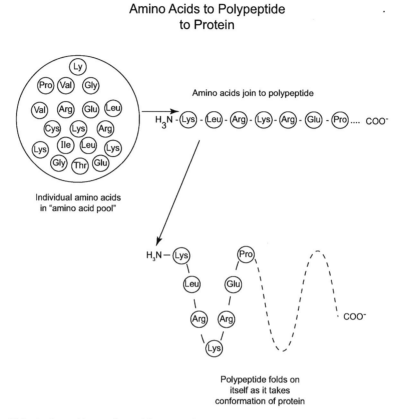

Fig. 13.3 Amino acids to polypeptide to protein

bonded together. The amino acids coded for on the mRNA must be available in the amino acid pool when their corresponding codon is read by the ribosome, or synthesis of that protein cannot progress. The amino acid pool is continuously replenished with new amino acids derived both from diet and stored proteins in the body in normal physiologic protein cycling.

Essential and Nonessential Amino Acids (Indispensable and Dispensable Amino Acids)

The amino acids are categorized into two groups, based on their dietary requirement, as either essential or nonessential. The essential, also termed indispensable, amino acids cannot be synthesized by humans. It is "essential" that they be obtained from dietary sources or stored body proteins (Table 13.1). The nonessential amino acids, also termed dispensable amino acids, can be synthesized by humans using

Protein Synthesis

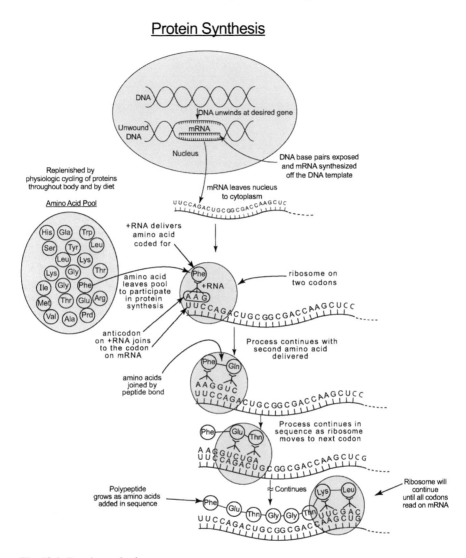

Fig. 13.4 Protein synthesis

other amino acids as substrate. Therefore, they do not have to be supplied by diet. It is important to understand that the terms essential and nonessential strictly refer to the body's ability to synthesize a specific amino acid from other amino acid precursors. All amino acids are critically important and irreplaceable in the proteins containing them that are used for the normal structure and function of the human body. Both categories could be termed "essential" in regard to importance in life.

The next series of terms for proteins, complete, incomplete, limiting, and complementary, are where I most often see confusion in patients. A food is termed a complete protein source if it contains all of the essential amino acids in

Table 13.1 The essential (indispensable) amino acids

Histidine
Threonine
Isoleucine
Tryptophan
Leucine
Valine
Lysine
Sulfur amino acids—methionine and cysteine
Aromatic amino acids—phenylalanine and tyrosine

the approximate ratio that the human body requires for protein synthesis. A food is termed an incomplete protein source if it contains one or more of the essential amino acids at a lower relative level than is necessary to approximate the ratio that the human body requires for protein synthesis. Complete proteins can, at absolute minimal protein intake levels, replenish all of the essential amino acid substrate pool "completely." Thus, in a theoretical scenario, if a complete protein, consumed at absolute minimal daily protein requirement levels, were the exclusive source for protein in the diet for a prolonged period of time, then there would still be an adequate dietary supply of essential amino acids. Incomplete proteins cannot, by themselves (if consumed at absolute minimum protein intake levels) replenish all of the essential amino acid substrate pool "completely." Incomplete proteins would "incompletely" supply one of the essential amino acids. Thus, in a theoretical scenario, if the only protein source in the diet for a prolonged period of time were an incomplete protein that was supplied at absolute minimal daily protein requirement levels, then there would ultimately be an inadequate supply of one of the essential amino acids. The terms "complete" and "incomplete" in describing proteins are not meant to synonymous with "good" and "bad." Rather, the terms are simply a way of citing the essential amino acid ratio in a food source. Indeed, nearly all protein-containing foods, grains, nuts, legumes, fish, eggs, dairy, and meat, irrespective of amino acid ratios, are sources for amino acids in the diet and are helpful to maintaining nitrogen balance in human nutrition.

The body cannot synthesize a protein if the amino acid pool is deficient in one of the amino acids contained in the desired protein. The missing amino acid is termed a "limiting amino acid," because its absence "limits" the body's ability to synthesize that protein that would otherwise be produced. However, in real-life scenarios, if a particular amino acid was low in the diet for a prolonged period of time, then the body would simply replete that amino acid in the pool from its stored supplies and normal synthesis would continue. Only with prolonged and severe malnutrition and consequent depletion of myriad storage structures would there truly be risk for a limiting scenario affecting health or body structure. The normal protein cycle in the body is designed so that catabolism of stored proteins will supply the amino acid pool as required.

Complementary protein sources are foods that by themselves contain incomplete proteins, but when combined they have the amino acid ratio of a complete protein source. In order to mimic a complete protein, a complemented protein source must have its relatively low amino acid increased to a higher absolute level. This occurs by the consumption of another protein source, the complementary source, which contains that amino acid in abundance. When considered as a single protein source, these combined foods now have the amino acid ratio of a complete protein and are said to "complement" one another. Protein complementation becomes relevant at prolonged, very low overall dietary protein intakes, at very low caloric levels, and in a vegan diet. In these scenarios, if complementary proteins are consumed either simultaneously or within a 24-h period of each other, their combined amino acids will continue to supply the amino acid pool with all of the essential amino acids at a level necessary for all protein synthesis. Otherwise, the body would rely on its stored amino acids to supply synthesis needs.

An example of complementing proteins can be described using grains as the protein source. Most grains have a relatively lower amount of lysine compared to their other amino acids. If a vegan consumed a diet of exclusively grains, he or she would eventually lack lysine in the amino acid pool. However, if beans or soy, which are rich in lysine, were consumed within a day of grain source proteins, these would "complement" the grain-amino acids and, together, mimic a complete protein. Also, any animal source protein such as egg whites, fat free dairy, or fish would "complement" the grain source in supplying the amino acid pool. In Table 13.2, the essential amino acid content of four protein sources is shown both as absolute amounts in mg/g of protein and as relative amounts (relative to World Health Organization recommended minimums) [1]. Note that lysine in whole-wheat flour is its limiting protein and that it would be complemented to far exceed WHO minimal requirements by any of the other protein sources.

From a dietary knowledge standpoint, the aforementioned terms and concepts are important to understand as they are often used in the lay press and arise in discussions with patients regarding diets of reduced animal product consumption, vegetarianism, and veganism. However, the terms complete, incomplete, limiting, and complementary proteins are only relevant to an individual's overall nutritional status if he or she severely restricts total caloric intake or only consumes foods nearly exclusively from a single plant source for a prolonged period of time. Otherwise, from a practical nutrition standpoint, nearly any combination of plant-based, whole food sources consumed in a balanced diet of adequate calories will result in abundant dietary essential and total amino acids to supply the amino acid pool. If any animal source proteins, egg whites, fat free dairy, fish, or lean poultry, are consumed, then it is essentially impossible to not meet all amino acid needs. In another way of looking at this issue, these numbers and descriptive terms would be important if one were managing patients on extreme, low-calorie diets (<800 cal/day) and trying to calculate what the absolute minimum protein requirement would be to achieve nitrogen balance. At absolute minimal energy and protein intake, any relative imbalance between the amino acid pattern of the diet and of the body's requirements becomes important whereas the identical pattern at a higher consumption level is irrelevant.

Table 13.2 Complete and incomplete proteins

	Milligram of essential amino acids per gram of protein				
	WHO minimum	Egg: % minimum	Black beans: % minimum	Whole wheat flour: % minimum	Salmon: % minimum
Histidine	15	24 → 160	28 → 187	27 → 180	29 → 193
Isoleucine	30	53 → 177	44 → 146	34 → 113	46 → 153
Leucine	59	86 → 146	80 → 136	68 → 115	81 → 137
Lysine	45	72 → 160	69 → 153	Limiting 27 → 60	92 → 204
Methionine and cysteine	22	52 → 236	24 → 110	38 → 173	40 → 182
Phenylalanine and tyrosine	30	94 → 313	82 → 273	72 → 240	73 → 243
Threonine	23	44 → 191	42 → 182	28 → 122	44 → 191
Tryptophan	6	13 → 216	12 → 200	13 → 217	11 → 183
Valine	39	68 → 174	52 → 133	43 → 110	51 → 131

Sources: World Health Organization (WHO) [1], US Department of Agriculture (USDA) nutrient data library [6]

Note: Egg and salmon significantly exceed World Health Organization (WHO) minimal percentages for every essential amino acid per gram of protein. They are complete protein sources

Black beans also exceed WHO minimal percentages, but only slightly for the sulfur amino acids methionine and cysteine

Whole wheat flour has one limiting amino acid: lysine. It is an incomplete protein source. Any of the other foods in the table would complement whole wheat flour

Daily Protein Requirement

Daily protein requirement is a measure of the amount of protein, as a mix of amino acids, which must be consumed to supply the metabolic demand of the body. Daily protein requirement may be represented qualitatively by Fig. 13.5.

To the extent that any of the daily protein requirement involves essential amino acids, this can only be met in the long run through dietary sources. However, over shorter periods of time that might be encountered, such as a 3-day fast, stored amino acids are mobilized from the tissues and organs to meet metabolic demands. In a moderately active individual, daily protein requirement is 15–20% of total calories in a 2,000 calorie diet. The World Health Organization puts the number at 0.83 g/kg/day [1]. In endurance athletes, I advise a daily

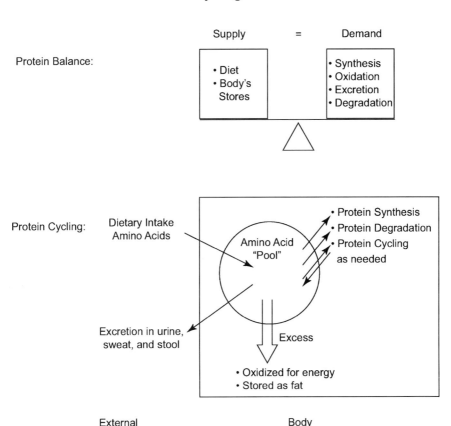

Fig. 13.5 Protein cycling and balance

intake of up to 1.2 g/kg/day. Calculated in grams per day at various body weights, the minimum daily protein requirements for adults and endurance athletes are shown in Table 13.3.

It is a common, but incorrect, assumption that any excess protein consumption will either stimulate extra muscle formation or will be stored as protein in the body for future usage. As with the carbohydrate and fat macronutrient classes, any protein consumption that exceeds the body's daily energy and synthesis requirements is ultimately converted to fat for storage. Chapter 9 on weight loss and control discusses how macronutrient balance does not affect obesity and body composition in greater detail.

In a Dietary Guidelines for Americans Committee (DGAC) 2010 analysis of three different variations of a Mediterranean-style diet for ability to meet protein requirement, all three far exceeded needs [2]. The first diet analyzed was termed "plant-based" with decreased amounts of meats and poultry and increased amounts of processed soy products, cooked dry beans and peas, and nuts so that 50% of all protein was plant-based. This diet mimics a traditional MedDiet, and was calculated to supply 177% of protein requirements. The second diet was a vegetarian diet termed "lacto-ovo" with elimination of all meats, poultry, and fish, and increased amounts of soy products, cooked dry beans and peas, nuts, and, to a lesser extent, eggs. This diet was calculated to supply 166% of protein requirements. The third diet was termed "vegan" with elimination of all animal products including meats, poultry, fish, eggs, milk and milk products, and increased amounts of soy products, cooked dry beans and peas, and nuts and seeds. This diet was calculated to supply 146% of protein requirements. These numbers demonstrate that diverse permutations of a healthy diet will all easily meet protein requirements (Table 13.4).

Author's Note

My goal is not to promote a vegetarian diet. I am not a vegetarian, nor is the MedDiet a vegetarian diet (although it can be if desired). The recipes and meal plans listed in this book contain delicious, healthy protein sources. Many do not contain any animal products, but many do as well. It is up to patients to decide what they choose to eat in this diet based on flavor and desire. I have taken care of ensuring the meals and recipes provide robust macronutrients at adequate levels from all classes and are excellent for health. If patients are interested in learning more about a vegetarian, semi-vegetarian diet, or reduced meat diet, then reliable Web sites to direct them to are:

The Vegetarian Resource Group: http://www.vrg.org/; also, http://www.vrg.org/nutrition/protein.htm [3].
The Vegetarian Society: https://vegsoc.org/ [4].
Medline plus: http://www.nlm.nih.gov/medlineplus/vegetariandiet.html [5].

Table 13.3 Safe level of protein intake for moderately active adults and for endurance athletes

Body weight		Safe level of protein intake (0.83 g/kg/day) calories[a,b]		Percent of total daily calories[c]			
		Protein gram (endurance athletes at 1.2 g/kg/day)	Protein calories	% of 1,000 cal	% of 1,500 cal	% of 2,000 cal	% of 2,500 cal
kg	lb						
50	110	42 (60)	168 (240)	17% (24)	11% (18)	8% (12)	7%
55	121	46 (66)	184 (264)	18% (26)	12% (20)	9% (14)	7%
60	132	50 (72)	200 (288)	20% (29)	13% (22)	10% (15)	8%
65	147	54 (78)	216 (312)	22% (32)	14% (24)	11% (16)	9%
70	154	58 (84)	232 (336)	23% (34)	15% (26)	12% (17)	9%
75	165	62 (90)	248 (360)	25%	17% (28)	12% (18)	10% (14)
80	176	66 (96)	264 (384)	26%	18% (30)	13% (19)	11% (15)
85	187	71 (102)	284 (408)	28%	19% (32)	14% (20)	11% (16)
90	198	75 (108)	300 (432)	30%	20% (34)	15% (22)	12% (17)
95	209	79 (114)	316 (456)	32%	21%	16% (23)	13% (18)
100	220	83 (120)	332 (480)	33%	22%	17% (24)	13% (19)
110	242	91 (132)	364 (528)	36%	24%	18% (26)	15% (21)

[a]World Health Organization (WHO)

[b]Safe level is 1–1.2 g/kg/day in endurance athletes (1:30 or greater exercise per day or greater than 10 h/week)

[c]Note that at lower total daily calories the absolute protein requirement in mg is unchanged, but it increases as a percentage of total calories

Table 13.4 Protein content of common Mediterranean diet foods

	Food	Protein/100 g	Protein cal/100 g
○	Peanuts	25.8	104
○	Peanut butter (smooth, no salt)	25.1	101
▬	Salmon	22	88
○	Almonds	21.2	85
○	Almond butter	21	84
▬	Trout, rainbow	20	80
▬	Halibut (cooked)	18.6	75
•	Tempeh	18.5	75
▬	Chicken (roast, light meat, cooked)	15.8	64
○	Walnuts	15.2	61
☐	Bread, whole wheat	10.9	44
▲	Egg whites	10.9	44
•	Kidney beans (cooked)	9.2	37
•	Lentils (cooked)	9.1	37
•	Pinto beans (cooked)	9	36
•	Black beans (cooked)	8.9	36
☐	Whole wheat pasta (cooked)	5.3	22
•	Tofu	4.8	19
☐	Quinoa (cooked)	4.4	18
☐	Amaranth (cooked)	3.8	16
▲	Milk, skim	3.4	14
▲	Milk, soy	2.9	12

Source: www.nal.usda.gov/fnic/foodcomp

References

1. Report of a Joint WHO/FAO/UNU Expert Consultation. Protein and amino acid requirements in human nutrition. WHO technical report series number 935;2002. http://whqlibdoc.who.int/trs/WHO_TRS_935_eng.pdf.
2. Dietary Guidelines for Americans Advisory Committee (DGAC) 2010. U.S. Department of Agriculture. Center for Nutrition Policy and Promotion. Dietary guidelines for Americans, 2010. http://www.cnpp.usda.gov/dietaryguidelines.htm. Accessed 1 Jan 2011.
3. The Vegetarian Resource Group. http://www.vrg.org/; http://www.vrg.org/nutrition/protein.htm. Accessed 27 May 2011.
4. The Vegetarian Society. https://vegsoc.org/. Accessed 27 May 2011.
5. Medline plus. http://www.nlm.nih.gov/medlineplus/vegetariandiet.html. Accessed 27 May 2011.
6. U. S. Department of Agriculture Nutrient Data Laboratory. www.nal.usda.gov/fnic/foodcomp. Accessed 27 May 2011.

Chapter 14
Alcohol

Keywords Mediterranean diet • Alcohol • Ethanol • Moderate consumption • Coronary heart disease • Alzheimer's disease • Stroke • Hypertension • Diabetes • Cancer

Moderate alcohol consumption is considered to contribute favorably to health in a Mediterranean diet. In MedDiet studies, "moderate alcohol consumption" is defined as 5–25 g of ethanol/day in women and 10–100 g/day in men. Figure 14.1 shows the volumes of 12% ethanol wine, 5% ethanol beer, and 40% ethanol (80 proof) distilled spirits that fit within this range. The United States Department of Agriculture (USDA) refers to "number of drinks" in its guidelines, defining "moderate alcohol consumption" as up to one drink per day for women and two drinks per day for men [1]. This USDA range, with each drink containing 17.75 g of ethanol, falls within the range of alcohol consumption considered favorable in a MedDiet (Fig. 14.2).

Any discussion of the health benefits of alcohol must emphasize that it is only potentially beneficial to health when three criteria are met: (1) consumed by adults, (2) consumed in moderation, and (3) consumed in controlled situations (i.e., not prior to driving an automobile, operating heavy or dangerous machinery, or handling a firearm or other weapon). Although alcohol misuse is an important cause of morbidity and mortality in our society, its consumption is also an integral part of our culture and, when consumed appropriately, it is a source of enhanced social pleasure, increased enjoyment of meals, and reduced cardiovascular disease (CVD) risks.

Because of the many risks associated with alcohol consumption, particularly excess consumption, no major health organization has ever called for encouraging nondrinkers to start consuming alcohol for their health. The general consensus is that if a mature adult regularly consumes alcoholic beverages in moderation, then he

E. Zacharias, *The Mediterranean Diet: A Clinician's Guide for Patient Care*, DOI 10.1007/978-1-4614-3326-2_14, © Springer Science+Business Media, LLC 2012

Moderate Alcohol Intake,
Mediterranean Diet Studies

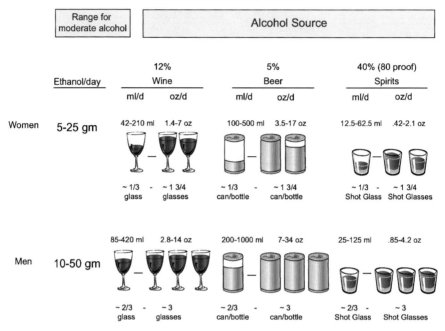

Fig. 14.1 Moderate alcohol consumption within the range of a MedDiet-adherence score (MedDiet-AS)

or she should be educated about the health effects of continued consumption, but people who do not drink should not be encouraged to start drinking since the potential CVD benefits are not overwhelmingly more favorable than the potential risks. Lastly, since each gram of alcohol provides 7 cal of energy, the liquid calories of alcoholic beverages can be a significant source of excess calories in the diets of individuals attempting to control their weight (Table 14.1) [2].

Perspective on the general positive and negative health consequences of alcohol as a single dietary variable on specific disease processes can be obtained from the following summaries.

Coronary Heart Disease

Numerous trials and review papers have reported that individuals who drink moderately have a lower risk of coronary heart disease (CHD) than nondrinkers. These effects are most often attributed to ethanol's effects on HDL-c, glucose, vasorelaxation, and clotting factors. Relative risk may be reduced by 15–40%. However, heavy or binge drinking increases risk of CHD [1, 3–7].

Moderate Alcohol Intake,
USDA Guidelines

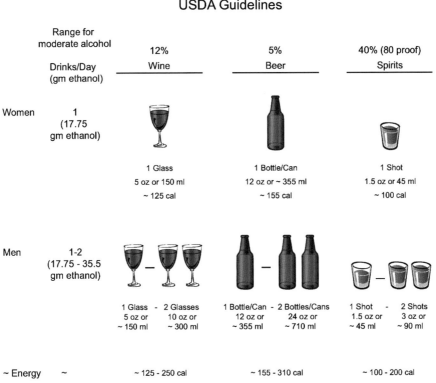

Fig. 14.2 USDA guidelines for moderate alcohol consumption

Table 14.1 Calories contained in one serving per type of alcoholic beverage

Common beverage	Common serving size	Energy in calories
80-Proof spirits	1.5 oz, 45 mL	100
Regular beer	12 oz, 355 mL	155
Wine	5 oz, 150 mL	125
Light beer	12 oz, 355 mL	100
Pina Colada	9 oz	500
Gin and tonic	6.5 oz	150
Margarita	6 oz	250
Mojito	6 oz	150
Martini	3 oz	250
Rum and Cola	6.5 oz	150
Screwdriver	6.5 oz	170
Whiskey sour	3.5 oz	160

USDA reference nutrient database [2]

Alzheimer's Dementia and Cognitive Impairment

Moderate alcohol consumption has been associated with a slower rate of cognitive decline with aging and reduced incidence of Alzheimer's disease. Heavy or binge drinking worsens both [1].

Stroke

Moderate alcohol consumption has been shown to reduce risk of stroke whereas heavy consumption increases risk [3, 8–13].

Hypertension

Moderate alcohol consumption does not increase risk of hypertension. However, heavier consumption increases hypertension [12, 14].

Diabetes

Moderate alcohol consumption increases insulin sensitivity, reduces fasting glucose levels, and decreases risk of type 2 diabetes (T2D) by up to 55% whereas heavy consumption increases T2D risk [15–17].

Cancer

At a moderate or greater level of consumption, alcohol increases risk for cancer of the colon, breast, and liver [18].

Total Mortality

Moderate alcohol consumption is associated with an approximately 20% reduction in all-cause mortality [19]. This overall mortality benefit derives from significant reduction in the common diseases of CHD, stroke, diabetes, and dementia that are prevalent in middle-aged and older men and women [20, 21].

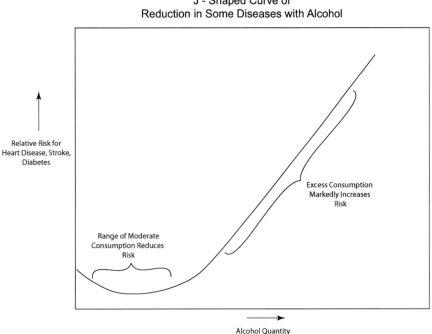

Fig. 14.3 J-shaped curve showing reduction in some diseases resulting from moderate alcohol consumption

Thus, since diseases of aging such as CHD, strokes, and dementia become more likely as an individual grows older, the relative health benefits of alcohol consumption become greater the older one is relative to the risks. In adults, when the mortality benefits of alcohol graphed, they are often described as appearing as a "J-shaped curve" (Fig. 14.3). This graphing reveals that some alcohol consumption is slightly better than none, but too much is markedly worse than moderate amounts or none at all.

Does the Source of the Ethanol Matter?

A common question is whether there is a "best" source for alcohol among wine, beer, and distilled spirits. Reviews of the large numbers of studies addressing this question note that there is no consistent evidence showing any advantage of one source over the others. Wine, beer, and distilled spirits, at equivalent grams of alcohol, show the same effects and should be considered equivalent in this regard [1, 22].

References

1. Dietary Guidelines for Americans Advisory Committee (DGAC) Dietary guidelines for Americans 2010, U.S. Department of Agriculture. Center for Nutrition Policy and Promotion; 2010. http://www.cnpp.usda.gov/dietaryguidelines.htm. Accessed 1 Jan 2011.
2. U.S. Department of Agriculture Nutrient Data Laboratory. www.nal.usda.gov/fnic/foodcomp. Accessed 27 May 2011.
3. Mukamal KJ, Jensen MK, Grønbaek M, Stampfer MJ, Manson JE, Pischon T, et al. Drinking frequency, mediating biomarkers, and risk of myocardial infarction in women and men. Circulation. 2005;112(10):1406–13.
4. Koppes LL, Twisk JW, Van Mechelen W, Snel J, Kemper HC. Cross-sectional and longitudinal relationships between alcohol consumption and lipids, blood pressure and body weight indices. J Stud Alcohol. 2005;66(6):713–21.
5. Solomon CG, Hu FB, Stampfer MJ, Colditz GA, Speizer FE, Rimm EB, et al. Moderate alcohol consumption and risk of coronary heart disease among women with type 2 diabetes mellitus. Circulation. 2000;102(5):494–9.
6. Muntwyler J, Hennekens CH, Buring JE, Gaziano JM. Mortality and light to moderate alcohol consumption after myocardial infarction. Lancet. 1998;352(9144):1882–5.
7. Booyse FM, Pan W, Grenett HE, Parks DA, Darley-Usmar VM, Bradley KM, et al. Mechanism by which alcohol and wine polyphenols affect coronary heart disease risk. Ann Epidemiol. 2007;17(5 Suppl):S24–31.
8. Bazzano LA, Gu D, Reynolds K, Wu X, Chen CS, Duan X, et al. Alcohol consumption and risk for stroke among Chinese men. Ann Neurol. 2007;62(6):569–78.
9. Emberson JR, Shaper AG, Wannamethee SG, Morris RW, Whincup PH. Alcohol intake in middle age and risk of cardiovascular disease and mortality: accounting for intake variation over time. Am J Epidemiol. 2005;161(9):856–63.
10. Elkind MS, Sciacca R, Boden-Albala B, Rundek T, Paik MC, Sacco RL. Moderate alcohol consumption reduces risk of ischemic stroke: the Northern Manhattan Study. Stroke. 2006;37(1):13–9.
11. Iso H, Baba S, Mannami T, Sasaki S, Okada K, Konishi M, et al. Alcohol consumption and risk of stroke among middle-aged men: the JPHC Study Cohort I. Stroke. 2004;35(5):1124–9.
12. Reynolds K, Lewis B, Nolen JD, Kinney GL, Sathya B, He J. Alcohol consumption and risk of stroke: a meta-analysis. JAMA. 2003;289(5):579–88.
13. Sundell L, Salomaa V, Vartiainen E, Poikolainen K, Laatikainen T. Increased stroke risk is related to a binge-drinking habit. Stroke. 2008;39(12):3179–84.
14. Taylor B, Irving HM, Baliunas D, Roerecke M, Patra J, Mohapatra S, et al. Alcohol and hypertension: gender differences in dose-response relationships determined through systematic review and meta-analysis. Addiction. 2009;104(12):1981–90.
15. Shai I, Wainstein J, Harman-Boehm I, Raz I, Fraser D, Rudich A, et al. Glycemic effects of moderate alcohol intake among patients with type 2 diabetes: a multicenter, randomized, clinical intervention trial. Diabetes Care. 2007;30(12):3011–6.
16. Baliunas DO, Taylor BJ, Irving H, Roerecke M, Patra J, Mohapatra S, et al. Alcohol as a risk factor for type 2 diabetes: a systematic review and meta-analysis. Diabetes Care. 2009;32(11):2123–32.
17. Howard AA, Arnsten JH, Gourevitch MN. Effect of alcohol consumption on diabetes mellitus: a systematic review. Ann Intern Med. 2004;140:211–9.
18. Di Castelnuovo A, Rotondo S, Iacoviello L, Donati MB, De Gaetano G. Meta-analysis of wine and beer consumption in relation to vascular risk. Circulation. 2002;105(24):2836–44.
19. Di Castelnuovo A, Costanzo S, Bagnardi V, Donati MB, Iacoviello L, de Gaetano G. Alcohol dosing and total mortality in men and women: an updated meta-analysis of 34 prospective studies. Arch Intern Med. 2006;166(22):2437–45.
20. Smith-Warner SA, Spiegelman D, Yaun SS, van den Brandt PA, Folsom AR, Goldbohm RA, et al. Alcohol and breast cancer in women: a pooled analysis of cohort studies. JAMA. 1998;279(7):535–40.

21. WCRF/AICR. Food, nutrition, physical activity, and the prevention of cancer: a global perspective. Washington, DC: AICR; 2007.
22. Mukamal KJ, Conigrave KM, Mittleman MA, Camargo Jr CA, Stampfer MJ, Willett WC, et al. Roles of drinking pattern and type of alcohol consumed in coronary heart disease in men. N Engl J Med. 2003;348(2):109–18.

Part V
Adopting a Mediterranean Diet

Chapter 15
Goal Is Success in Adoption

Keywords Mediterranean diet • Healthy eating • Diet substitutions • Diet additions

The remainder of this book is designed to help patients successfully adopt a Mediterranean diet. This section chiefly presents ways to make long-term healthy eating as convenient as unhealthy eating. For example, patients in my clinic often note a lack of time for preparing healthy meals as well as not having the building block ingredients on hand at home for preparing healthy food. They then resort to the most readily available, generally unhealthy, foods. This section contains information to help overcome these and other barriers including examples of quick on-the-go meals for the time pressed; an extensive number of delicious and healthy Mediterranean recipes, and meal ideas that may be used for nearly any meal scenario; and a detailed shopping list for helping to maintain healthy food staples stocked at home. Internet resources that provide quality recipes and reliable information about eating for health are also listed.

An important step to take when helping with practical implementation of a MedDiet is to ensure that patients have a solid understanding of the diet's principal components. A summary of these follows:

Principal components of a Mediterranean diet
High intake of plant foods that are minimally processed and seasonally fresh. This includes vegetables, fruits, unrefined cereals and bread, beans, legumes, nuts, and seeds
Plant oils as primary source of dietary fat, particularly olive oil and canola oil
Moderate to low intake of dairy products, consumed chiefly as low-fat yogurt and cheese
Moderate to low intake of poultry and low to very low intake of red meat and processed meat and meat products
Weekly or greater consumption of fish
Less than four egg yolks per week
Infrequent consumption of concentrated sweets
Daily alcohol, usually wine, in low to moderate amounts and generally with meals

E. Zacharias, *The Mediterranean Diet: A Clinician's Guide for Patient Care*,
DOI 10.1007/978-1-4614-3326-2_15, © Springer Science+Business Media, LLC 2012

Once patients understand a MedDiet's constituent nutrients, they are then in a position to review information for its practical implementation including food substitutions and additions, eating on the go, and food in social situations. The figures and descriptions that follow are designed to show patients that eating a MedDiet requires easily implemented dietary approaches.

Substitutions, Additions

Food substitutions and additions are two easy strategies that can transform foods common in a Western diet into ones more consistent with a MedDiet. "Substitutions" is a technique to reduce or eliminate unfavorable nutrients by substituting healthy ingredients for the less healthy ones (such as substituting olive oil for butter in a recipe). "Additions" is a technique to increase favorable nutrients by adding healthy MedDiet ingredients (such as adding beans or vegetables to pasta dishes) to foods. Reviewing the tables and figures that follow with patients can simplify the process of teaching them about using substitutions and additions to improve the health quality of their diets:

Table 15.1 shows both the more and the less MedDiet style foods in different major food categories. The goal is to substitute the foods in the "More Mediterranean Style" category for the foods in the "Less Mediterranean Style" category when purchasing or preparing foods.

Figure 15.1 shows examples of "MedDiet friendly foods" that can be added to common foods. The goal is, when practical, to add these ingredients when purchasing or preparing foods.

Table 15.2 applies the information from Table 15.1 and Fig. 15.1 to a few common Western diet foods and meals to show how they can be made more consistent with a MedDiet.

On the Go, Med-Enough

An important area I address with patients is how they can adhere to a MedDiet when time and convenience are paramount in their lives. In my practice many patients note that time pressures, not lack of intellectually understanding what they should ideally be eating, result in their consuming unhealthy foods. Patients report when hungry they find it too difficult to quickly prepare or find healthy food so they resort to the most convenient (frequently unhealthy) option. Over the years I have developed lists of foods for these patients that contain the essence of a MedDiet's favorable, health-promoting characteristics and are also very quick to prepare or find as well as being highly portable. One particularly important part of using this strategy requires the patient to organize on the front end their pantry, freezer, and refrigerator

Table 15.1 Ingredient and food substitutions to make foods more consistent with a Mediterranean diet

Less Mediterranean style	Substitute with	More Mediterranean style
Grains/breads/cereals		
White bread	→	Whole wheat and whole multigrain bread
White rice	→	Brown rice, quinoa
White pasta	→	Whole wheat pasta
White flour in baking	→	1/2 white and 1/2 whole wheat flour
Processed flour cereals	→	Whole grain cereals
Fruits/vegetables		
Sweetened fruits and juices	→	Naturally unsweetened fruits and juices
Baked potatoes	→	Seasoned roasted or steamed vegetables, brown rice, quinoa
Oils/fats		
Butter	→	Extra virgin olive oil
Shortening	→	Extra virgin olive oil, canola oil
Partially hydrogenated margarines	→	Extra virgin olive oil, nonhydrogenated margarines
Meats/animal protein sources		
Steak	→	Fish steaks or filets, skinless chicken breasts
Hamburgers, ground beef	→	Veggie burgers, fish burgers, "mock meats"
Cold cuts	→	Lean sliced turkey or chicken
Sausage, hotdogs, meat products	→	Meat substitute products, "mock meats"
Whole eggs	→	Egg whites, egg substitute
Beverages		
Regular soda	→	Diet soda, water with lemon or lime, unsweetened tea or coffee
Whole fat milk	→	Fat-free milk, soy, or almond milk
Sports drinks	→	Water with lemon or lime, 1/2 strength diluted with water
Snacks and other foods		
Potato chips	→	Apple slices, mixed nuts
Ice cream	→	Fat-free sugar-free frozen yogurt, fruit with fat-free plain yogurt
Cream-based dips	→	Hummus, guacamole
Sour cream	→	Fat-free plain or Greek yogurt
Sugar	→	Use half in recipes, use noncaloric sweetener
Regular crackers	→	Whole grain crackers
High volumes of cheese	→	Low volumes of intense flavor cheese such as goat cheese, feta, parmesan, gruyere, bleu, extra sharp cheddar
Most desserts	→	Fruit with yogurt or nut butters; small piece of dark chocolate

Additions to Make Any Food More Mediterrean

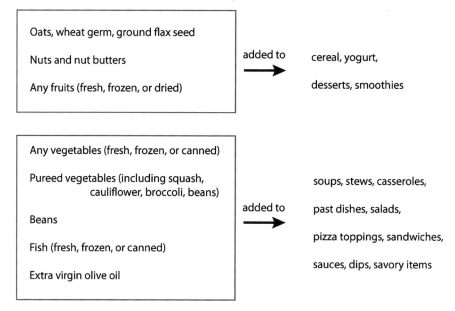

Fig. 15.1 MedDiet-friendly additions to common foods

Table 15.2 Examples of substitutions and additions to common foods to make them more consistent with a Mediterranean diet

Less consistent with a MedDiet	More consistent with a MedDiet
Breakfast-type foods	
Processed, sweetened cereal with 2% milk	Whole grain cereal, unsweetened nuts and raisins added, with skim, soy, or almond milk
Tall glass orange juice	Tall glass 1/2 water and 1/2 orange juice or water with squirt lemon or lime juice
White flour pancakes or waffles	Whole wheat or multigrain flour pancakes or waffles, topped with fruit and chopped nuts
Bacon or sausage side	Meatless sausage or bacon substitute
Whole egg omelet cooked in butter	Egg white or egg substitute omelet cooked in extra virgin olive oil
Lunch-type foods	
White bread sandwich with roast beef and cheese	Whole wheat bread sandwich with lean turkey, tuna, or hummus and sliced avocado
Potato chips	Baby carrots, celery, or grape tomatoes, mixed nuts
Cookie	Apple, orange, or grapes
Entrée-type foods	
White flour tortilla burrito with ground beef, cheese, and sour cream	Whole wheat flour burrito with black beans, sautéed onions and green peppers, and guacamole
Teriyaki beef on white rice	Teriyaki tofu on brown rice with mixed vegetables
Hamburger on white bun	Veggie or salmon burger on whole grain bun
Steak and potato	Salmon, halibut, or other fish steak or filet and quinoa salad

Table 15.3 "Mediterranean enough" meal ideas for patients on the go

Breakfast	Lunch and dinner	Snacks
Cereal mix to tumbler with fruit and nuts	Whole grain crackers or bread with nut butters	Trail mix
Oatmeal with fruit and nuts	Salad bar at grocery, quick serve	Fruit ± added nut butters
Egg white or substitute scramble on whole wheat toast	Whole grain bread sandwich with hummus, nut butter, turkey, tuna	Mixed nuts
Fruit smoothie	Smoothie	Hummus with baby carrots or whole grain crackers
Banana with almond or peanut butter	Pressed fruit and nut bar with nut butters	See breakfast items
Whole grain toast with olive oil or nut butter	Can vegetable soup plus can beans	1 or 2 squares dark chocolate
Hard-boiled eggs, yolk removed	Microwaved veggie, salmon, or tuna burger on whole wheat toast	Olives
Cup of yogurt with fruit slices and/or nuts	Microwaved whole wheat flour tortilla burrito	Toasted whole wheat or multigrain bun plus olive oil
	Any leftover re-served	
	Falafel balls	

to keep them well stocked with healthy ingredients and prepared foods. Patients may be directed to and encouraged to use the grocery list as a way to keep ingredients on hand and easily usable so they can optimize the MedDiet quality of their daily food intake. I tell patients that these suggestions are designed to "Americanize" the convenience and speed side and "Mediterraneanize" the nutrition side of quick meals. I term this fashion of healthy eating "Mediterranean Enough." It is understandable that patients may be pressed for time and unable to enjoy leisurely prepared, multi-ingredient foods, but it need not be inevitable that time pressures result in their consuming unhealthy foods.

The "Mediterranean Enough" series of recommendations that follow show how to consume healthy foods in time-pressed situations, and they closely mirror what I eat when I am very busy at work or at home. Although there are days where one might want to escape their stress and relax with fine foods and wine, the reality of a busy American life is that this is often not possible. People generally eat food three or more times daily and limiting MedDiet-consistent meals only when time and situation allow is not often enough to receive the full benefits of the diet, particularly if the alternative food consumed is of an unhealthy nature. Table 15.3 shows MedDiet style foods to eat for health when time is limited.

Bringing Food

Food is an integral part of social interaction in nearly all cultures, and it is important to address with patients how MedDiet food can be a part of common social situations. The "Recipes" section of this book provides dozens of selections that are appropriate for use as entrees, sides, appetizers, and desserts in nearly any social scenario. The examples in Tables 15.4–15.6 demonstrate the use of MedDiet foods for a few common scenarios and may be used by patients exactly as written or may be used to stimulate creativity.

Table 15.4 Examples of Mediterranean diet-consistent foods for a school party (see Chap. 18 for recipes)

Fruit crisp
Chocolate pudding
Chilled yogurt fruit salad
Fruit and granola parfaits
Multigrain carrot muffins
Granola banana muffins

Table 15.5 Examples of Mediterranean diet-consistent foods for a sports event potluck (see Chap. 18 for recipes)

Roasted eggplant and walnut dip
Whole bean dip
Spiced mix nuts
Guacamole
Hummus
Zesty walnut hummus
Black bean and goat cheese quesadilla
Smoked salmon quesadilla
Herb-roasted vegetables
Simple roasted squash
Quinoa salad with agave-mint dressing
Mediterranean quinoa salad
Salsa

Table 15.6 Examples of
Mediterranean diet-consistent
foods to stock in a corporate
break room

Fruits
  Bananas
  Apples
  Oranges
  Grapes
  Seasonal fruit
Vegetables
  Baby carrots
  Cherry or plum tomatoes
  Celery stalks
  Cauliflower florets
  Broccoli florets
Dips and spreads
  Hummus
  Peanut butter
  Almond butter
Bread
  Whole wheat and multigrain bread
Nuts
  Mixed nuts
Yogurt
  Individual plain yogurts
Beverages
  Lemon and lime squeeze bottles for
    adding to water
  Coffee
  Tea
  Soy or almond milk
  Fat-free dairy

Chapter 16
Meal Plans

Keywords Mediterranean diet • Meal plans • Weight control

Structuring an easy to set-up and follow meal plan may assist patients in their efforts to lose and control weight with a MedDiet. One effective way to do this is to show patients how to arrange the meals and foods they find appealing within the diet in a fashion that is easy to visualize, follow, and modify. The steps that this entails and an example of a structured meal plan follow. Importantly, when a patient is using a MedDiet for weight loss, they should be instructed that they do not need to deprive themselves of any of the delicious foods contained in the diet. However, they do need to practice moderation in their portions at meal time and to minimize or eliminate between-meal snacking (see Chap. 9 for more information on dieting for weight loss). Table 16.1 should be referenced when discussing the following steps:

Step 1: Create meal options for each day and place in the appropriate column. The number of meal options may be increased over time as additional appealing meals are discovered.

Step 2: Consume exclusively one option from each column each day. Portion sizes should be moderate and no other caloric sources should be consumed. Drinking extra water is encouraged. Record what was consumed in a daily food and activity log.

Step 3: If after about 3 weeks weight is not declining, then the portion size of each meal option should be reduced by about 20% and physical activity should remain the same or increase.

Step 4: Review and repeat Step 3 as many times as necessary until weight loss is steady at 1–4 lb per month. If desired weight loss is not occurring, patients should do an honest, self-critical assessment for extra caloric intake that they are not recording.

E. Zacharias, *The Mediterranean Diet: A Clinician's Guide for Patient Care*,
DOI 10.1007/978-1-4614-3326-2_16, © Springer Science+Business Media, LLC 2012

Table 16.1 Examples of Mediterranean diet meals structured for weight loss and control (see also Chap. 15, Table 15.3)

Breakfast options	Lunch options	Dinner options	Snack options
Cereal, grab and go[a] Beverages[b]	Salmon or black and white bean burger on wholegrain bun[a] Apple, orange, or grapes Baby carrots Beverages	Pistachio dill salmon on wild rice[a] Fava bean salad[a] Beverages (optional 1 glass wine)	Trail mix[a]
Smoothie[a] Beverages	Mediterranean chicken salad, curried chicken salad, or tuna/salmon salad on whole wheat bread[a] Apple, orange, or grapes Baby carrots Beverages	Paella[a] Beverages (optional 1 glass wine)	Hummus with vegetables[a]
Hearty whole-grain waffle or pancakes[a] Beverages	Veggie, bean, and hummus pita[a] Apple, orange, or grapes Baby carrots Beverages	Smoked salmon quesadilla[a] Beverages (optional 1 glass wine or beer)	Spiced mixed nuts[a]
Mixed vegetable frittata[a] Beverages	Subway® 6-in. veggie patty Sandwich on whole grain bread, no cheese, multiple veggie toppings, low calorie sauce Apple slices Beverages	Fennel, white bean, and walnut salad[a] Whole grain bread with extra virgin olive oil Beverages (optional 1 glass wine or beer)	Banana, apple, orange, grapes or other fruit ± nut butter
Ultimate oatmeal[a] Beverages	Hearty lentil and brown rice soup[a] Baby carrots, celery, or tomatoes with hummus (premade or see Chap. 18 recipes)	Seafood stew[a] Whole grain bread with extra virgin olive oil Beverages (optional 1 glass wine or beer)	Quick yogurt cup[a]
Toast with egg and avocado[a] Beverages	Smoothie[a] Beverages	Spaghetti with marina and vegetables[a] Beverages (optional 1 glass wine or beer)	2 Squares dark chocolate

Chocolate toast[a]	Mediterranean quinoa salad[a]	Herb-roasted vegetables[a]	Multigrain carrot muffin[a]
Beverages	Beverages	Carrot and ginger soup[a]	
		Beverages (optional 1 glass wine or beer)	
Quick yogurt cup[a]	Beverages = same as breakfast	Beverages = same as breakfast	Snack options or any of the meal options may be consumed all at once or divided throughout the day
Beverages			

[a]See Chap. 18 for recipes

[b]Beverages = large glass water ± splash lemon or lime juice. Optional: coffee or tea ± skim milk ± sweetener

Step 5: Once a healthy, desired weight is achieved, maintain the caloric intake (portion sizes and meals) and activity levels that have achieved this balance.

Step 6: Understand that there is a 100% chance of regaining lost weight if a positive energy balance occurs either through increasing caloric intake or reducing activity. Alternatively, there is a 100% chance that weight will remain stable when a neutral energy balance occurs or will decrease further with a negative energy balance.

As a final summation of using a MedDiet for weight loss, providers may remind patients that the body is an infallible calorie-counting machine. Lifelong awareness of body weight, caloric consumption, and activity levels may be of benefit in losing weight. As long as they consume fewer calories than they burn, thus achieving a negative energy balance, they will lose weight. Table 16.1 and the outlined steps may be used as a way to track consumption and may assist with weight loss and control. Patients must understand that excess caloric consumption will inevitably result in weight gain.

Chapter 17
Shopping List, Keep On Hand

Keywords Mediterranean diet • Grocery list • Vegetables • Fruit • Nuts • Seeds
• Oils • Breads • Fish • Meat • Meat substitutes • Cereals • Dairy • Eggs • Condiments
• Pasta • Beans • Beverages • Baking

A well-stocked and organized supply of Mediterranean diet-friendly foods at home can facilitate healthy eating. Over the years, I have found one of the most common causes of dietary noncompliance at home is patient inattention to the logistics of shopping. The goal of using the grocery list that follows is to keep the home well stocked, easy, and consuming healthy foods at home, a convenient dietary choice.

E. Zacharias, *The Mediterranean Diet: A Clinician's Guide for Patient Care*,
DOI 10.1007/978-1-4614-3326-2_17, © Springer Science+Business Media, LLC 2012

Grocery List

Fresh Vegetables

- [ ] Artichoke
- [ ] Avocado
- [ ] Arugula
- [ ] Asparagus
- [ ] Basil (fresh)
- [ ] Broccoli
- [ ] Beets
- [ ] Bell peppers
- [ ] Carrots
- [ ] Cabbage
- [ ] Cauliflower
- [ ] Chard
- [ ] Celery
- [ ] Corn
- [ ] Cucumber
- [ ] Eggplant
- [ ] Garlic
- [ ] Ginger
- [ ] Green beans
- [ ] Hot peppers
- [ ] Herbs (fresh)
- [ ] Kale
- [ ] Lettuce
- [ ] Leeks
- [ ] Mushrooms
- [ ] Olives
- [ ] Onions
- [ ] Parsley
- [ ] Peas
- [ ] Peppers—green, red
- [ ] Potatoes
- [ ] Salad greens
- [ ] Spinach
- [ ] Sprouts
- [ ] Squash
- [ ] Sweet potatoes
- [ ] Tomato
- [ ] Zucchini
- [ ] _____

Fresh Fruit

- [ ] Apples
- [ ] Apricots
- [ ] Bananas
- [ ] Blackberries
- [ ] Berries
- [ ] Blueberries
- [ ] Cantelope
- [ ] Cherries
- [ ] Cranberries
- [ ] _____

Dried Fruits

- [ ] Fig/dates
- [ ] Grapes
- [ ] Grapefruit
- [ ] Kiwi
- [ ] Lemons
- [ ] Limes
- [ ] Melon
- [ ] Mangoes
- [ ] Oranges
- [ ] Peaches
- [ ] Pears
- [ ] Pineapple
- [ ] Plums
- [ ] Pomegranate
- [ ] Prunes
- [ ] Raspberries
- [ ] Watermelon
- [ ] _____
- [ ] _____

Nuts and Seeds/Nut Butters

- [ ] Almonds
- [ ] Brazil nuts
- [ ] Cashews
- [ ] Hazelnuts
- [ ] Peanuts
- [ ] Pecans
- [ ] Pine nuts
- [ ] Pistachios
- [ ] Pumpkin
- [ ] Sunflower
- [ ] Walnuts
- [ ] _____

Nut Butters

- [ ] Peanut butter
- [ ] Almond butter
- [ ] Squeeze packs
- [ ] Trail mix
- [ ] Snacks
- [ ] _____

Frozen Fruits and Vegetables

Vegetables

- [ ] Broccoli
- [ ] Corn
- [ ] Spinach
- [ ] Vegetable medley
- [ ] Others
- [ ] _____

Fruit

- [ ] Blueberries
- [ ] Mixed berries
- [ ] Strawberries
- [ ] Others

Canned Items/Canned Vegetables and Fruits

Vegetables

Beans

- [ ] Baked
- [ ] Black
- [ ] Chickpeas/garbanzo
- [ ] Fava
- [ ] Kidney
- [ ] Lentils
- [ ] Lima
- [ ] Pinto
- [ ] White
- [ ] Carrots
- [ ] Corn
- [ ] Garlic
- [ ] Green beans
- [ ] Olives
- [ ] Peas
- [ ] Pickles
- [ ] Tomatoes
- [ ] Vegetable broth
- [ ] _____

Fruit

- [ ] Apple sauce
- [ ] Peaches
- [ ] Pears
- [ ] Pineapple
- [ ] Tangerine
- [ ] Other fruits
- [ ] _____

Other Canned

- [ ] Salmon
- [ ] Soups
- [ ] Tuna

- [ ] Others
- [ ] _____
- [ ] _____

Oils

- [ ] Extra virgin olive oil
- [ ] Canola oil
- [ ] Sesame oil
- [ ] Spray nonstick oil
- [ ] _____

Breads

- [ ] Whole grain bread
- [ ] Multi-grain bread
- [ ] Whole grain bagels
- [ ] Whole wheat tortillas
- [ ] Whole wheat pitas
- [ ] Whole wheat English muffins
- [ ] Whole grain buns
- [ ] Whole grain crackers
- [ ] _____

Fish/Meat/Meat Substitute

- [ ] Chicken
- [ ] Turkey
- [ ] Sliced deli meat
- [ ] Meat substitute
- [ ] Tofu/vegetarian substitutes
- [ ] Breakfast meat substitutes
- [ ] Tempeh
- [ ] Tofu
- [ ] Fish
- [ ] Other seafood
- [ ] _____
- [ ] _____

Frozen Fish/Meat Substitutes/ Prepared
- ☐ Burritos
- ☐ Fish burgers
- ☐ Fish filets
- ☐ Veggie burgers, patties
- ☐ Prepared food
- ☐ _____

Cereals
- ☐ Whole grain flakes/squares
- ☐ Granola
- ☐ Multigrain cereals
- ☐ Oats
- ☐ Oatmeal
- ☐ Whole wheat pancake/waffle mix
- ☐ _____

Dairy/Cheese/Egg
- ☐ Fat-free milk
- ☐ Almond milk
- ☐ Soy milk
- ☐ Cottage cheese, fat free
- ☐ Sour cream, fat free
- ☐ Yogurt, fat free
- ☐ Yogurt, Greek
- ☐ Cheese
- ☐ Eggs
- ☐ Egg substitute/whites
- ☐ Margarine, non-hydrogenated
- ☐ _____
- ☐ _____

Condiments/Sauces
- ☐ Agave nectar
- ☐ BBQ sauce
- ☐ Brown rice syrup
- ☐ Honey
- ☐ Hot sauce
- ☐ Jelly and jam
- ☐ Ketchup
- ☐ Mayonnaise—canola or olive oil
- ☐ Mustard
- ☐ Pesto
- ☐ Salad dressing
- ☐ Salsa
- ☐ Soy sauce
- ☐ Sriracha
- ☐ Tabasco
- ☐ Tahini

Vinegars
- ☐ Balsamic
- ☐ Red wine
- ☐ White wine
- ☐ Others
- ☐ Worcestershire
- ☐ _____
- ☐ _____

Pasta, Dried Beans
Beans, dried
- ☐ Black
- ☐ Black-eyed peas
- ☐ Chickpeas
- ☐ Fava
- ☐ Kidney
- ☐ Lentil
- ☐ Lima
- ☐ Mixed

- ☐ Navy
- ☐ Peas
- ☐ Pinto
- ☐ White
- ☐ Couscous, whole grain
- ☐ Pasta, whole wheat
- ☐ _____

Beverages
- ☐ Alcohol
- ☐ Beer
- ☐ Wine
- ☐ Others
- ☐ Coffee
- ☐ Coffee filters
- ☐ Drink mixes
- ☐ Lemon juice
- ☐ Lime juice
- ☐ Tea
- ☐ Others
- ☐ _____

Baking
Grain Flours, Whole
- ☐ Amaranth
- ☐ Barley
- ☐ Brown rice
- ☐ Buckwheat
- ☐ Bulgur
- ☐ Corn meal
- ☐ Flax
- ☐ Millet
- ☐ Multigrain cereals

- ☐ Oats
- ☐ Quinoa
- ☐ Spelt
- ☐ Wheat berries
- ☐ Wild rice
- ☐ Others
- ☐ _____

Herbs and Spices
- ☐ Allspice
- ☐ Anise
- ☐ Basil
- ☐ Bay leaves
- ☐ Black pepper
- ☐ Cayenne
- ☐ Chives
- ☐ Cinnamon
- ☐ Cilantro
- ☐ Cloves
- ☐ Chili powder
- ☐ Coriander
- ☐ Cumin
- ☐ Curry powder
- ☐ Dill
- ☐ Fennel
- ☐ Garlic powder
- ☐ Garlic salt
- ☐ Marjoram
- ☐ Mustard powder
- ☐ Nutmeg
- ☐ Oregano
- ☐ Paprika
- ☐ Parsley
- ☐ Peppermint
- ☐ Poppy seeds
- ☐ Red pepper

- ☐ Saffron
- ☐ Sage

Salt
- ☐ Iodinated
- ☐ Kosher
- ☐ Sea
- ☐ Tarragon
- ☐ Thyme
- ☐ Turmeric
- ☐ Vanilla
- ☐ Others
- ☐ _____

Other Baking
- ☐ Baking powder, Al-free
- ☐ Baking soda
- ☐ Brown sugar
- ☐ Chocolate
- ☐ Cocoa
- ☐ Sugar
- ☐ Sugar substitutes
- ☐ Sweeteners
- ☐ Yeast
- ☐ Other
- ☐ _____
- ☐ _____

Chapter 18
Resources

Keywords Mediterranean diet • Recipes • Food products • Vegetarian • Books • Movies • Web sites

This section lists resources that can be accessed for further information on eating for health.

Recipes/Food Products

When searching for recipes on Web sites, seek ones that adhere to the principles of a MedDiet as outlined in Chap. 15 "Principal Components of a Mediterranean Diet." The following Web sites either sell products that fit well into a MedDiet or have a database of searchable recipes that may be modified as desired using the techniques of food substitutions and additions as discussed in Chap. 15, section "Substitutions, Additions" (see Fig. 15.1 and Tables 15.1 and 15.2 for examples).

Oldwayspt.org: This organization promotes the health benefits of a MedDiet. The Web site contains useful information regarding the diet and a searchable collection of MedDiet recipes.

http://topics.nytimes.com/top/news/health/series/recipes_for_health/index.html: The *New York Times* has this searchable recipe database that provides hundreds of healthy recipes.

Bobsredmill.com: A great source that sells virtually every whole grain product that exists. I use their products in baking and in meal preparation to increase my variety and quantity of whole grains. Their Web site has a searchable database of hundreds of healthy recipes for all occasions.

Aboutseafood.com: A good source for searchable seafood recipes of all varieties.

E. Zacharias, *The Mediterranean Diet: A Clinician's Guide for Patient Care*,
DOI 10.1007/978-1-4614-3326-2_18, © Springer Science+Business Media, LLC 2012

Epicurious.com: An enormous database of searchable recipes.

http://www.montereybayaquarium.org/cr/cr_seafoodwatch/download.aspx; http://www.nrdc.org/oceans/seafoodguide/; and www.edf.org/seafoodhealth: These are three sites with reliable information about which seafood is most sustainable: a point that is important to some patients in making decisions about what to purchase.

Fruitsandveggiesmorematters.com: This promotional site for produce contains a large number of ideas and recipes that can help patients incorporate more fruits and vegetables into their diets.

Justinsnutbutters.com: a company that solved the issue of how to make healthy and versatile nut butters more portable through their clever use of single-serving squeeze packages.

Walnuts.org: This site has numerous recipes using walnuts, one of the healthiest of all nuts.

Vegetarianism

As noted before, a MedDiet is not necessarily a vegetarian diet, but it does emphasize a more plant-based diet than is typical in a Western diet. Additionally, vegetarian diets are generally very easy to adapt to fit the definition of a MedDiet (see Chap. 15, "Principal Components of a Mediterranean Diet."). These sites contain reliable information for patients who desire to research vegetarianism or who wish to learn more about increasing plant-based foods in their omnivorous diet further:

The Vegetarian Resource Group: http: //www.vrg.org/; also, http: //www.vrg.org/nutrition/protein.htm

The Vegetarian Society: https: //vegsoc.org/
Medline plus: http: //www.nlm.nih.gov/medlineplus/vegetariandiet.html

Books

The following books provide interesting reading for patients who wish to read investigative journalist-style books about America's food sources and dietary habits. They are not about a MedDiet per se, but they share a theme with a MedDiet of reducing simple and refined sugars, processed foods, and animal fats while increasing plant-based foods in the diet to improve health outcomes.

The Omnivores Dilemma, by Michael Pollan

In Defense of Food: *An Eater's Manifesto*, by Michael Pollan

Animal, Vegetable, Miracle: *A Year of Food Life*, by Barbara Kingsolver

Fast Food Nation: *The Dark Side of the All-American Meal*, by Eric Schlosser

Eating Animals, by Jonathan Foer

Movies

I love the fact that movies are being made that attempt to call the attention of large audiences to the importance of a healthy diet. These movies have different styles, but they all ultimately attempt to improve the eating patterns of Americans. They are not specifically about a MedDiet, but many of the important themes of a MedDiet are presented in an engaging fashion, and some patients may find it motivating to eat a better diet after watching these.

Food, Inc.: This engaging movie shows the corrupting influence of corporate factory farming on our food supply, and, ultimately, our health.

Fast Food Nation: A very good movie that makes a strong case for the corrupting influence of the fast food industry on American's health and obesity.

Supersize Me: This brilliantly conceived movie is simultaneously entertaining and disturbing as one man shows the effects of a poor diet on his health. I think it is a "must view."

Forks Over Knives: Probably the weakest of the four movies listed here, it still entertainingly presents the important theme that healthy eating can prevent many diseases.

Personal Web Sites

Mediterraneanenough.com: This is a Web site I created that speaks to patients in a casual fashion regarding some of the basics of a Mediterranean diet. In addition to general information on a MedDiet and its health effects, there is a blog section covering my time studying the diet while in the Mediterranean countries.

Zabbatical.com: This Web site contains my family's blog about our times living overseas when I was researching to write this book. There is also some information on how to take your family abroad for an extended family sabbatical.

Chapter 19
Recipes

Keywords Mediterranean diet • Recipes • Breakfast • Appetizers • Soups • Salads • Sides • Entrees • Desserts • Beverages

The heart of a Mediterranean diet is its delicious, health-promoting foods. Patients can use the compilation of recipes that follows for their daily meals, for special occasions, and for nearly any conceivable dining situation. For purposes of organization, the recipes are categorized as breakfast, appetizers, soups, salads and sides, entrees, desserts, and beverages.

Recipe Categories

Appetizers

Roasted eggplant and walnut dip
White bean dip
Spiced mixed nuts

Breakfast

Hearty whole grain pancakes and waffles
Toast with egg and avocado
Ultimate oatmeal
Chocolate toast
Cereal grab and go

E. Zacharias, *The Mediterranean Diet: A Clinician's Guide for Patient Care*,
DOI 10.1007/978-1-4614-3326-2_19, © Springer Science+Business Media, LLC 2012

Bruschetta

Bruschetta with cannellini

Burger Alternatives

Salmon burger
Black and white burger

Chili

Red chili
White chicken chili

Curry

Single pan curry cauliflower

Desserts

Fruit crisp
Chocolate pudding
Chilled yogurt fruit salad
Fruit and granola parfaits

Fish

Maple salmon on wilted spinach
Pistachio dill salmon on wild rice
Italian white fish on quinoa
Sautéed fish Provencal

Frittata

Mixed vegetable frittata
Asparagus dill

Gazpacho

Gazpacho

Guacamole

Guacamole

Hummus

Hummus
Zesty walnut hummus

Muffins

Multigrain carrot muffins
Granola banana

Paella

Paella

Pasta

Whole wheat penne with garbanzos and spinach
Pesto and tomato
Marinara and veggies
Mediterranean pasta salad
Mediterranean lasagna

Pizza

Quick pita red or green

Quesadillas

Black bean and goat cheese
Smoked salmon

Ratatouille

Ratatouille

Roasted Vegetables

Roasted balsamic beets
Harvest vegetables with roasted ginger and cumin
Herb roasted vegetables
Simple roasted squash

Sandwich, Wraps, Pita

Veggie, bean, and hummus pita
Veggie wrap
Tuna/Salmon salad wrap/sandwich

Salad (Green)

Greens and tuna

Salad (Meat/Fish)

Mediterranean chicken salad
Curried chicken salad
Tuna/salmon salad

Salad/Sides (Vegetable)

Lentil carrot
Green bean salad with walnuts
Wild rice, asparagus, and pecan
Brown and wild rice, walnuts, and dried cranberry
Roasted chickpeas and spinach
Couscous salad with chickpeas, dates, and cinnamon
Foreign legion
Lentil salad
Fava bean salad
Artichoke-oregano-antipasti
Fennel, white bean, and walnut salad
Eggplant caponata
Butternut squash and beans

Salad (Quinoa)

Quinoa salad with agave-mint dressing
Mediterranean quinoa salad

Salsa

Salsa

Smoothie

Smoothie options

Soups/Stews

Carrot and ginger soup
Hearty lentil and brown rice soup
Three bean soup
Seafood stew
Pasta e fagioli

Stir Fry

Ginger carrot stir-fry
Broccoli stir-fry

Recipe Names by Food Category

Categories

1. Appetizers and snacks
2. Breakfast
3. Entrees
4. Soups and stews
5. Salads and Sides
6. Desserts

Arugula salad: 5
Avocado salsa: 1
Bean salad: 5
Broccoli stir fry with tofu or chicken: 3
Brown and wild rice, California walnuts, and dried cranberry salad: 5
Bruschetta with cannellini: 1
Carrot and ginger soup: 4
Cereal ready to grab and go: 2
Chilled fruit and yogurt bowl: 1, 6
Chocolate toast: 2
Curried cauliflower with peas and carrots: 3
Curried tuna salad: 5
Fennel, white bean, and walnut salad: 5
Fruit, granola, and yogurt parfaits: 6
Gazpacho: 4
Granola morning muffins: 2
Green bean salad with walnuts: 5
Guacamole: 1
Herb roasted vegetables: 5
Hummus: 1
Italian white fish: 3
Lentil and brown rice soup: 4
Maple salmon on wilted spinach: 3
Mediterranean chicken salad: 5
Mediterranean quinoa salad: 5
Mixed vegetable frittata: 2

Multigrain pancakes or waffles: 2
Multigrain carrot muffins: 2
Oatmeal: 2
Paella: 3
Pasta fagioli: 3
Pesto: 1
Pistachio dill salmon: 3
Pita pizzas: 1, 3
Quesadillas with goat cheese and black bean: 1, 3
Quinoa salad with mint and lime: 5
Red chili with three beans: 4
Roasted balsamic beets: 5
Rustic tuna on greens: 5
Salmon burgers: 3
Sautéed fish provencal: 3
Savory mixed nuts: 1
Seafood stew: 4
Simple fruit crisp: 6
Smoked salmon and asparagus frittata: 2
Smoked salmon quesadilla: 1, 3
Smoothies, multiple options: 1, 2
Spaghetti with vegetables and chicken or tofu: 3
Three bean Italian soup: 4
Toast with egg and avocado: 2
Tofu: How to cook: 3
Trail mix: 1
White bean dip: 1
White chili with chicken: 4

Appetizers and Snacks

Avocado Salsa

Serves 4–6

Ingredients

1 can (15 oz or 425 g) shoe peg or regular corn, drained
5 Roma tomatoes, diced
1 Medium red onion, chopped
2 Ripe avocados, peeled, pitted, and diced

½ Green bell pepper, seeded and diced
1 Clove garlic, minced
¼ Cup (60 mL) fresh cilantro, chopped
1 tbsp (15 mL) red wine vinegar
2 tbsp (30 mL) extra virgin olive oil
3 tbsp (45 mL) lime juice
¼ tbsp ground cayenne pepper
½ tbsp (2.5 mL) sea or kosher salt
½ tbsp (2.5 mL) coarsely ground black pepper

Directions

1. Combine all ingredients in a medium-sized bowl and mix until evenly distributed.
2. Serve with corn chips or as a festive topping for salad.

Notes

This salsa is a nutritious appetizer served with whole grain corn chips, woven whole wheat crackers, carrots, cauliflower, or red bell pepper slices. It may also be used as a topping for fish filets or whole wheat tortilla burritos.

Bruschetta with Cannellini

Serves 4–6

Ingredients

1 Whole grain or multigrain baguette cut on the diagonal into approximately ½ in. (2.5 cm) slices
1 Can (about 15.5 oz or 425 g) cannellini beans, well drained
½ Cup (125 mL) plus 1 tbsp (15 mL) extra virgin olive oil
3 Medium tomatoes, finely chopped
½ Cup (125 mL) freshly grated parmesan cheese
2 Cloves garlic, minced
¼ Cup (60 mL) coarsely chopped fresh basil leaves
½ tbsp dried oregano
¼ Cup balsamic vinegar
¼ tbsp (1.25 mL) kosher or sea salt

Directions

1. Place bread on baking sheet, brush with ½ cup (125 mL) olive oil and toast in oven preheated to 400°F (220°C) until golden brown.
2. In medium bowl, mix tomatoes, garlic, basil, oregano, 1 tbsp olive oil, balsamic vinegar, parmesan, and cannellini beans until evenly mixed.
3. Spoon mixture onto bread slices and serve immediately.

Notes

One may make variations of this dish by substituting crumbled feta cheese for the parmesan cheese and/or rosemary leaves for the basil leaves. This dish is most often served as an appetizer or as part of a tapas dinner. For a variation, this same recipe may be used to make a flavorful bean salad side dish.

Chilled Fruit and Yogurt Bowl

Serves 8

Ingredients

6 Cups (1,500 mL) of assorted fruits of choice—including banana, blackberries, blueberries, cantaloupe, kiwi, mango, raspberries, seedless grapes, strawberries—sliced or cubed
2 Cups (500 mL) fat-free plain yogurt
2 tbsp (30 mL) orange juice
2 tbsp (30 mL) lemon juice
1 tbsp (5 mL) poppy seeds
¼ tbsp (1.25 mL) ginger
½ tbsp nutmeg
Optional: ¼ cup (60 mL) shredded coconut

Directions

1. In medium bowl, mix orange juice, lemon juice, poppy seeds, ginger, and nutmeg. Then add yogurt and stir until blended.
2. In large bowl, place fruit and then gradually add yogurt mix while stirring gently to evenly coat fruit.
3. Refrigerate for 1 h and serve chilled.

Notes

This dish is great as a healthy dessert alternative and can be served in casual or more formal dishes depending on the situation. It is also great for picnics, potlucks, and keeping in the refrigerator as a quick snack. Doubling or tripling the recipe in an extra large bowl allows for nutritious sides, desserts, and snacks for several days.

Guacamole

Ingredients

4 Avocados, halved and seeded
2 tbsp (30 mL) lime juice
2 tbsp chopped cilantro leaves
1 Medium tomato, cored and diced
1 Small onion, chopped
2 Cloves garlic, minced
½ tbsp (2.5 mL) cumin
¼ tbsp (1.25 mL) chili powder
½ tbsp (2.5 mL) cayenne
½ tbsp (2.5 mL) kosher or sea salt
Optional: add 1 small can, about 7 oz (200 g) of corn kernels, well drained

Directions

1. Scoop pulp from avocados and place in medium bowl. Add lime juice and mash the avocados.
2. Add remaining ingredients and mixing until evenly distributed.

Notes

This is a straightforward recipe for guacamole. In addition to being delicious when served with chips, guacamole may be used as a dip for vegetable platters and as a spread for a variety of sandwiches and burgers.

Hummus

Serves 4

Ingredients

1 Can (15 oz or 425 g) garbanzo beans, drained with liquid reserved
½ Cup (125 mL) tahini
¼ Cup (60 mL) lemon juice
2 Cloves garlic, chopped
2 tbsp (5 mL) cumin
½ Cup (125 mL) olive oil
¼ tbsp (1.25 mL) kosher or sea salt
¼ tbsp (1.25 mL) ground black pepper

Directions

1. In food processor or blender, add all ingredients. Blend ingredients until even consistency, adding reserved liquid as needed to make creamier.

Notes

This is a typical hummus recipe that may be made more spicy with cayenne or crushed red pepper if desired. Hummus is great served with a vegetable tray including celery, baby carrots, cherry or plum tomatoes, and sliced cucumber. It is also a flavorful spread for a variety of sandwiches.

Pesto

Yields 1½ cups (375 mL)

Ingredients

4 Cups (1,000 mL) packed fresh basil leaves
3 Cloves garlic
⅓ Cup (85 mL) pine nuts, very lightly toasted (may substitute walnuts) just before using
⅔ Cup (170 mL) extra virgin olive oil
½ Cup (125 mL) grated parmesan cheese
Kosher or sea salt and fresh ground black pepper to taste.

Directions

1. In a blender or food processor combine basil, garlic, and very lightly toasted pine nuts (or walnuts) and pulse until basil is chopped. You will have to stop pulsing frequently to push basil down to initial chop.
2. Once basil mixture is evenly chopped add olive oil, pulse until smooth, and pour into a bowl. Next, add the Parmesan cheese, salt, and pepper and stir until smooth.
3. Serve immediately.

Notes

Pesto is one of my favorite Mediterranean foods. It can be tossed with nearly any pasta dish, used as a spread on sandwiches, wraps, and quesadillas, or used as a dip for bread or vegetables.

Pita Pizzas: Red or Green

Serves 4

Ingredients

Both:

6 Large whole wheat pita rounds
2 tbsp (30 mL) extra virgin olive oil

For Red

1 Can (about 6.5 oz or 190 mL) tomato sauce
1 Red bell pepper, chopped
½ Cup (120 mL) crimini mushrooms, halved
1 Onion, diced
8–10 Kalmata olives, quartered (may substitute marinated artichoke quarters)
½ tbsp dried basil
½ tbsp dried oregano
½ Cup (125 mL) mozzarella cheese
¼ Cup (60 mL) grated parmesan cheese
Optional: 6 marinated artichoke hearts, quartered

For Green

⅔ Cup (160 mL) pesto sauce
1 Cup (250 mL) cherry or grape tomatoes, halved
10–12 Kalmata olives, halved (may substitute marinated artichoke quarters)
½ Cup (120 mL) crimini mushrooms, halved
1 Can (15 oz or 425 g) white beans, well drained
6 oz (170 g) goat cheese, crumbled

Directions

1. Preheat oven to 425°F (220°C).
2. Place pita rounds on baking sheets and top evenly with olive oil, then top with sauce (pesto or red)
3. Add respective toppings and bake 10 min.

Notes

These flavorful quick pizzas can serve as appetizers or meals. The toppings can be modified based on personal tastes and ingredients on hand.

Quesadillas with Goat Cheese and Black Bean

Serves 4

Ingredients

4 Whole wheat tortillas
2 tbsp (10 mL) extra virgin olive oil
1 Can (15 oz or 425 g) black beans, well drained
1 Red bell pepper, chopped
1 Medium onion, chopped
1 Ripe avocado, sliced lengthwise
½ Cup (250 mL) cilantro, chopped
½ Cup (125 mL) goat cheese

Directions

1. Assemble quesadilla by dividing ingredients evenly on 2 tortillas, then top each with remaining tortillas.

2. In large non-stick skillet add oil and turn on medium heat. Cook one quesadilla at a time for about 3–4 min each side until slightly brown.
3. Cut into wedges and serve.

Notes

Quesadillas are a quick to prepare and nutritious choice for appetizers or whole meals. Scrambled or fried egg whites/egg substitute may be added to make these breakfast quesadillas.

Savory Mixed Nuts

Yield 5 cups

Ingredients

5 Cups (1,250 mL) shelled, unsalted, mixed nuts (may include almonds, walnuts, hazelnuts, cashews, peanuts, and shelled pistachios)
½ Cup (125 mL) extra virgin olive oil
½ tbsp (2.5 mL) sea salt or kosher salt
2 tbsp (5 mL) garam masala
½ tbsp (2.5 mL) ground cayenne pepper

Directions

1. Preheat oven to 325°F (165°C).
2. Place nuts in large bowl, pour in olive oil, and stir to coat. Gradually add salt, garam masala, and cayenne to nuts while stirring to coat.
3. Spread mixture on baking sheet lined with aluminum foil and bake for 10 min, removing once to mix after about 5 min.
4. Place roasted nuts on thick layer of paper towels to absorb excess oil, and serve once cooled.

Notes

Spiced nuts are a great appetizer or snack, and they are a nice addition to potlucks and picnics.

Smoked Salmon Quesadilla

Serves 4

Ingredients

4 Whole wheat tortillas
4 oz (110 g) smoked salmon
2 tbsp (10 mL) extra virgin olive oil
2 tbsp (30 mL) capers
1 Ripe avocado, peeled, seeded, and sliced lengthwise
1 Red onion, sliced
12 Cherry or plum tomatoes, halved
½ Cup (125 mL) goat cheese

Directions

1. Assemble quesadilla by dividing ingredients evenly on 2 tortillas and then topping each with remaining tortillas.
2. In a large non-stick skillet add oil and turn on medium heat. Cook one quesadilla at a time for about 3–4 min each side until slightly brown.
3. Cut into wedges and serve.

Notes

These flavorful quesadillas combine several classic MedDiet ingredients in a quick to prepare and nutritious choice for appetizers or whole meals. Scrambled or fried egg whites/egg substitute may be added to make these breakfast quesadillas.

Smoothies, Multiple Options

Serves 1–4

Ingredient Options

Berries/Fruits	Liquids	Additional ingredients
Ripe banana	Skim milk	Rolled oats
Strawberries	Soy milk	Peanut butter
Blackberries	Almond milk	Almond butter
Blueberries	Orange juice	Whey protein powder
Mango	Apple juice	Soy protein powder
Peaches	Yogurt	Shredded coconut
Pears	Ice	Granola topping
Pineapples		
Blackberries		
Watermelon		
Raspberries		
Apple sauce		

Directions

1. Combine desired ingredients from each category in blender in quantity to make volume of smoothie wanted. Blend until smooth adding liquid or ice as needed.
2. Serve immediately.

Notes

A smoothie can serve as a great breakfast, lunch, or snack option. Experiment with different combinations based on interests and ingredients on hand. With a well-stocked refrigerator and pantry (see Chapter 17 Grocery List) smoothies can always be ready within just a few quick minutes.

Trail Mix

Ingredients

1 Cup (250 mL) peanuts
1 Cup (250 mL) almonds
½ Cup (125 mL) shelled sunflower or pumpkin seeds
½ Cup (125 mL) raisins
½ Cup (125 mL) other dried fruit
Optional: 1 cup (250 mL) granola, ½ cup (125 mL) dark chocolate chips, ¼ cup (60 mL) shredded coconut

Directions

1. Combine all ingredients in large bowl and mix together. Store in airtight food containers or plastic food bags.

Notes

Trail mix is a healthier alternative to most snacks. There are an infinite number of combinations of nuts, legumes, and dried fruits that may be tried to create one's own favorite mixes.

White Bean Dip

Ingredients

2 Cans (about 15 oz, or, 425 g, each) cannellini beans, drained
2 Cloves garlic
½ Cup (125 mL) extra virgin olive oil
1 tbsp (5 mL) rosemary
1 tbsp (5 mL) dried parsley
½ tbsp (2.5 mL) ground cumin
1 tbsp (5 mL) lemon juice
½ tbsp (2.5 mL) of sea salt or kosher salt
Ground black pepper

Directions

1. Blend the beans, garlic, lemon juice, and olive oil in blender or food processor until just smooth.
2. Gradually add rosemary, parsley, cumin, salt, and pepper while continuing to puree until evenly mixed.

Notes

This dip is delicious and versatile. It may be used as a traditional dip for corn chips, whole-wheat pita, and for mixed vegetables such as baby carrots, cherry tomatoes, sliced cucumber, and sliced red bell peppers. It may also be used as a spread served on bread with sandwiches or burgers.

Breakfast

Cereal Ready to Grab and Go

Ingredients to Keep Stocked and Easily Accessed in Pantry and Refrigerator

Large tub filled with mix of multigrain and whole grain cereals and granolas
Individual container with rolled oats
Individual container with walnuts and/or almonds
Bag of raisins
Bananas
Other fresh and frozen fruit
Skim, soy, or almond milk
Fat-free plain yogurt

Directions

1. Fill bowl or large volume cup, preferably with a handle, with 1 cup of cereal mix and ½ cup of rolled oats.
2. Add small handful of nuts and fruit or fruits of choice.
3. Add ½ cup of yogurt if desired and pour on milk.

Notes

This system is what I use at home for nearly every workday breakfast. It allows me to prepare a nutritionally complete and satisfying breakfast in under 1 min. Most mornings I prepare this in a large cup or tumbler with a handle and carry the cereal around, eating it while I am preparing for the day.

Chocolate Toast

Ingredients and Directions

1. Toast one slice per person of whole wheat bread or baguette
2. Spread thin layer of almond, peanut, or hazelnut chocolate butter (such as Justin's or other brand)
3. Drizzle approximately 1 tbsp of extra virgin olive oil on each slice

Notes

Chocolate toast can serve as a quick breakfast, snack, or meal substitute. For a less chocolaty flavor, one may spread half natural peanut butter or almond butter along with the chocolate nut butter.

Granola Morning Muffins

Yield 16 muffins

Ingredients

1 ½ Cup (375 mL) whole wheat pastry flour (Bob's Red Mill or other brand)
1 ½ Cup (375 mL) granola, flavor of choice
1 Cup (250 mL) apple sauce
½ Cup (125 mL) fat-free plain yogurt
1 Very ripe banana, mashed
½ Cup (125 mL) egg whites or egg substitute
3 tbsp (45 mL) extra virgin olive oil
1 tbsp (15 mL) baking powder
1 tbsp (5 mL) ground cinnamon
1 tbsp (5 mL) all spice
1 tbsp (5 mL) vanilla extract
½ tbsp (2.5 mL) kosher or sea salt
1 Cup (250 mL) chopped walnuts
Optional: 1 cup (250 mL) raisins (add more sweetness), or 1 cup (250 mL) dark chocolate chips

Directions

1. Preheat oven to 350 F (175 C).
2. In large mixing bowl, combine flour, granola, baking powder, cinnamon, all spice, salt, and walnuts and mix until blended.
3. In separate, medium mixing bowl add apple sauce, yogurt, banana, egg, olive oil, and vanilla and whisk together for about 1 min until of evenly blended and uniform consistency.
4. Pour wet ingredients into dry ingredients and gently fold in until evenly combined.
5. Pour batter into muffin tins sprayed liberally with non-stick spray and bake for 25 min. Remove, allow to cool, and serve.

Notes

This recipe is not for sweetened dessert cupcakes but for a healthy, semi-savory hybrid of muffins and scones—rich in fiber and whole grains. These muffins work nicely for breakfast or a nutritious snack when warmed by briefly microwaving or toasting and then spreading with a non-hydrogenated oil margarine (such as Smart Balance™) and fruit jam. A morning cup of coffee or tea makes enjoying the muffins even better.

Mixed Vegetable Frittata

Serves 4

Ingredients

1 Cup (250 mL) of egg whites or egg substitute
¾ Cup (185 mL) broccoli, chopped or ¾ cup (185 mL) thawed green peas
¾ Cup (185 mL) spinach, chopped
1 Red bell pepper, chopped
1 Medium onion chopped
2 Cloves garlic, minced
¼ Cup (60 mL) mushrooms, chopped
2 tbsp (30 mL) extra virgin olive oil
1 tbsp (2.5 mL) herbes de Provence
¼ tbsp (1.25 mL) sea or kosher salt
¼ tbsp (1.25 mL) ground black pepper
2 tbsp (30 mL) freshly grated Parmesan cheese

Directions

1. Add olive oil to medium sized non-stick, oven-proof skillet. Add onions and garlic and sauté over medium high heat for about 2 min. Add other vegetables, herbes de Provence, salt, and pepper, and continue to cook over medium heat for about 5 min while stirring frequently.
2. Reduce heat to medium and add eggs by pouring evenly over vegetables; then cook until eggs just begin to firm and add Parmesan cheese to top of eggs. Next, place skillet in oven about 8 in under broiler. Cook for about 5 min until eggs just begin to brown.
3. Remove skillet from oven and serve hot.

Notes

This frittata is equally popular for breakfast, brunch, lunch, or dinner. I usually make for breakfast and then re-heat leftovers whenever in the mood.

Multigrain Carrot Muffins

Yield 16 muffins

Ingredients

2 Cups (500 mL) whole wheat pastry flour
1 Cup (250 mL) grated carrot
1 Cup (250 mL) raisins
1 Cup (250 mL) 7, 10, or 12 grain hot cereal (such as from Bob's Red Mill)
½ Cup (125 mL) egg whites or egg substitute
½ Cup (125 mL) extra virgin olive oil or walnut oil
¼ Cup (60 mL) brown sugar
1 tbsp (15 mL) baking powder
1 tbsp (5 mL) cinnamon
2 tbsp (10 mL) nutmeg
1 tbsp (5 mL) allspice
½ tbsp ground cloves
½ tbsp kosher or sea salt
2 tbsp (10 mL) vanilla extract
1 Cup (250 mL) apple sauce
1 ½ Cup (375 mL) skim, soy, or almond milk
Optional: 1 cup (250 mL) chopped walnuts or dark chocolate chips

Directions

1. Preheat oven to 350°F (175°C). Spray muffin tins with non-stick cooking spray.
2. In large mixing bowl, combine flour, hot cereal, baking powder, cinnamon, nut-meg, allspice, cloves, salt, and optional nuts, and mix until evenly blended.
3. In separate mixing bowl combine carrot, egg, oil, brown sugar, apple sauce, vanilla, and milk. Whip these for about 1 min until even consistency.
4. Pour wet ingredients into dry and fold together until just evenly blended.
5. Pour batter into muffin tins and bake for 30 min until done.

Notes

These muffins are full of healthy vegetables, whole grains, plant oils, and fiber. Once baked, they are highly portable, and can serve as a complete breakfast, lunch, or snack. These also work well for potlucks.

Multigrain Pancakes or Waffles

Yield 4–5 waffles or 10–12 large pancakes.

Ingredients

2 Cups (500 mL) whole wheat flour (use whole wheat pastry flour for lighter waffles)
1 Cup (250 mL) old fashioned oats (rolled oats)
½ Cup (125 mL) 10-, or 12-grain hot cereal (Bob's Red Mill is a commonly available brand)
½ Cup (125 mL) wheat germ
1 tbsp (30 mL) baking powder
½ tbsp (2.5 mL) baking soda
½ tbsp (2.5 mL) kosher or sea salt
1 Cup (250 mL) chopped walnuts or pecans (optional)
½ Cup (125 mL) applesauce
1 Cup (250 mL) egg substitute or egg whites
¼ Cup (60 mL) extra virgin olive oil
1 ½ Cup (375 mL) skim, soy, or almond milk; if needed may add extra milk 1 tbsp (15 mL) at a time to maintain batter consistency
½ tbsp (2.5 mL) vanilla extract

Directions

1. Combine dry ingredients (flour, oats, cereal, wheat germ, baking powder, baking soda, salt, and nuts) in large bowl and mix to blend together. Next, add egg, olive oil, applesauce, and milk. Stir until batter reaches an even consistency and then gradually add any additional milk needed to reach proper "ladling" consistency.
2. Ladle batter onto non-stick griddle or waffle iron.

Notes

Pancakes or waffles may be topped with any combination of non-hydrogenated spread (such as Smart Balance™), maple syrup, fresh sliced bananas or fruit, or microwave-thawed frozen fruit. I make these waffles nearly every weekend for myself and anyone who happens to be around.

Oatmeal

Ingredients and Directions

1. Prepare 1–2 cups of oatmeal or multigrain hot cereal cooked with boiled water to desired consistency. (I prefer rolled and steel cut oats for their body).
2. As desired, mix in and top hot cereal with the following items:

- Chopped walnuts or pecans
- Fresh cut or thawed frozen berries
- Sliced banana
- Raisins
- Peanut butter or almond butter
- Skim, soy, or almond milk

Notes

Oatmeal is a great way to start the day. This recipe is a reminder to use creativity and experimentation with MedDiet ingredients using the cooked oatmeal as the base for any combination of healthy toppings and mix-ins. Try different combinations of the listed toppings and other nuts and fruits to find what you like.

Smoked Salmon and Asparagus Frittata

Serves 4

Ingredients

1 Cup (250 mL) of egg whites or egg substitute
¼ Pound (115 g) smoked salmon, sliced
1 Pound (450 g) asparagus stalks, cut into 1-in (2.5 cm) pieces
2 tbsp (30 mL) extra virgin olive oil
2 tbsp (10 mL) dried dill
½ tbsp (2.5 mL) tarragon
¼ tbsp (1.25 mL) ground black pepper
¼ tbsp (1.25 mL) sea or kosher salt to taste (use less if smoked salmon using is particularly salty)
¼ Cup (60 mL) feta cheese, finely crumbled

Directions

1. In a medium sized, ovenproof skillet, add olive oil and asparagus and heat over medium heat for about 3 min until stalks begin to soften. Then add dill, tarragon, salt, and pepper and stir gently for about 1 min.
2. Pour eggs over mixture and then immediately add the salmon and feta cheese, distributing evenly. Continue to cook uncovered until the eggs just begin to firm and then remove skillet from burner and place in oven on rack about 6 in under broiler. Broil for about 3–5 min or until top of eggs just begin to brown. Remove and serve.

Notes

This nutritious dish delivers gourmet flavor and is relatively quick to make. It is equally popular for breakfast, brunch, lunch, or dinner.

Smoothies, Multiple Options

Serves 1–4

Ingredient Options

Berries/Fruits	Liquids	Additional ingredients
Ripe banana	Skim milk	Rolled oats
Strawberries	Soy milk	Peanut butter
Blackberries	Almond milk	Almond butter
Blueberries	Orange juice	Whey protein powder
Mango	Apple juice	Soy protein powder
Peaches	Yogurt	Shredded coconut
Pears	Ice	Granola topping
Pineapples		
Blackberries		
Watermelon		
Raspberries		
Apple sauce		

Directions

1. Combine desired ingredients from each category in blender in quantity to make volume of smoothie wanted. Blend until smooth adding liquid or ice as needed.
2. Serve immediately.

Notes

A smoothie can serve as a great breakfast, lunch, or snack option. Experiment with different combinations based on interests and ingredients on hand. With a well-stocked refrigerator and pantry (see Chapter 17 Grocery List) smoothies can always be ready within just a few quick minutes.

Toast with Egg and Avocado

Serves 4

Ingredients

1 Baguette (whole grain) sliced lengthwise; (may substitute 4 slices of whole-grain bread)
2 Ripe avocadoes, peeled, pitted, and sliced lengthwise
2 Tomatoes, sliced
4 tbsp (60 mL) extra virgin olive oil
1 Cup (250 mL) egg substitute or egg whites
¼ tbsp (1.25 mL) sea or kosher salt
¼ tbsp (1.25 mL) coarsely ground black pepper

Directions

1. Drizzle olive oil on top of baguette or 4 slices of bread and broil until golden brown.
2. Cook eggs in non-stick pan.
3. Place eggs on toasted bread, top with tomato and avocado slices, sprinkle lightly with salt and black pepper to taste.

Notes

I love this recipe for a quick and nutritious breakfast loaded with MedDiet nutrients.

Entrees

Broccoli Stir Fry with Tofu or Chicken

Ingredients

12 oz. (340 g) boneless, skinless chicken breast, cubed, or 1 block firm tofu, cut into small cubes
2 Cups (500 mL) broccoli florets
½ Cup (125 mL) mushrooms, sliced
1 Carrot, chopped
1 Red bell pepper, chopped
3 tbsp (45 mL) ginger root, finely chopped (or use pre-chopped, jarred ginger)
½ Cup (125 mL) cilantro, chopped
3 Cloves garlic, minced (or use 1 tbsp [5 mL] pre-minced, jarred garlic)
3 tbsp (45 mL) canola oil

1 tbsp (15 mL) soy sauce
1 tbsp (15 mL) rice vinegar
1 tbsp (15 mL) toasted sesame seeds
½ tbsp (2.5 mL) sea or kosher salt
½ tbsp (2.5 mL) ground black pepper
Optional: 1 red onion, diced; 1 cup (250 mL) toasted, unsalted cashews

Directions

4. In large skillet or wok, heat oil over medium high heat for about 3 min while swirling frequently. Add chicken or tofu (see section "Tofu: How to Cook") and cook for about 2 min, stirring frequently. Reduce heat to medium and add remainder of ingredients while stirring continuously for about 5 min.
5. Turn off heat and serve immediately.

Notes

This recipe contains a great combination of MedDiet ingredients flavored in a more Asian style. It may be served alone, but I usually serve it over brown rice or quinoa and often double the recipe for leftovers as it reheats well.

Curried Cauliflower with Peas and Carrots

Serves 4

Ingredients

1 Cauliflower, cut into florets (about 2 lb or 1,800 g)
2 Cups (500 mL) frozen peas
2 Medium carrots, peeled and cubed
1 Large onion, chopped
4 Cloves garlic, minced
2 tbsp extra virgin olive or canola oil
1 Can (about 15 oz or 425 g) stewed tomatoes (may substitute diced tomatoes)
2 tbsp (30 mL) curry powder
2 Cups (250 mL) vegetable stock
1 tbsp garam masala
¼ tbsp (1.25 mL) cayenne (reduce to just a pinch if a less spicy version is desired)
½ tbsp (2.5 mL) kosher or sea salt

Optional: 1-pound skinless chicken breast or tofu (see "Tofu, how to cook"), cubed and sautéed in olive or canola oil over medium high heat until browned.

Directions

1. Using large skillet, heat canola oil over medium high heat and sauté onion and garlic in canola oil. Once starting to brown, add vegetable stock and can of stewed tomatoes.
2. Add remainder of ingredients (including optional tofu or chicken) and spices while gently stirring and bring to boil.
3. Reduce heat to medium low and simmer covered for 30 min stirring occasionally and add additional pinches of salt to taste. Serve over brown rice or quinoa.

Notes

This relatively quick to make curry dish contains the nutritional essence of MedDiet in a dish typical of a different ethnic region. It is a nice complement to the more traditional Mediterranean-region flavors. Double the dish for extra leftovers as this dish reheats very well for several days.

Italian White Fish

Ingredients

2 Pounds (900 g) skinned white fish fillets such as cod, hake, halibut, or sole
1 Green bell pepper, chopped
1 Yellow bell pepper, chopped
1 Medium onion, chopped
1 Can (about 15 oz or 425 g) stewed tomatoes
6 Kalmata olives, seeded and quartered
6 Medium-sized green olives, seeded and quartered
2 tbsp (30 mL) extra virgin olive oil
3 Cloves garlic, minced
1 tbsp (15 mL) capers
1 tbsp (15 mL) lime juice
½ tbsp (2.5 mL) kosher or sea salt
½ tbsp ground black pepper

Directions

1. Preheat oven to 350°F (175°C).
2. In nonstick skillet, place olive oil, onion, and garlic and sauté over medium high heat until just starts to brown. Reduce heat to medium and add bell peppers. Heat for another 3 min, then add stewed tomatoes, olives, and capers. Cover and simmer for approximately 10 min.
3. While the sauce is simmering, place fish in a shallow casserole dish liberally sprayed with nonstick spray. Drizzle lime juice over fish and sprinkle with salt and pepper. Bake at 350°F (175°C) until just flaky and remove.
4. Pour contents of skillet over fish in casserole dish and then serve immediately.

Notes

This flavorful fish dish is complemented by many of the recipes in this chapter served as side items including arugula salad, brown and wild rice salad, bean salad, fennel salad, Mediterranean quinoa salad, quinoa salad with mint and lime, herb roasted vegetables, roasted beets, and roasted squash.

Maple Salmon on Wilted Spinach

Serves 4–6

Ingredients

2 Pounds (900 g) of salmon fillets
1 Pound (450 g) spinach

Marinade:

¼ cup (60 mL) extra virgin olive oil
¼ cup (60 mL) maple syrup
¼ cup (60 mL) soy sauce
2 cloves garlic, minced
2 tbsp (10 mL) sesame seeds
1 tbsp (5 mL) orange juice
1 tbsp (15 mL) paprika
½ tbsp (2.5 mL) cayenne
1 tbsp chili powder
¼ tbsp sea or kosher salt

Directions

For Salmon and Marinade:

1. Combine all of marinade ingredients in medium bowl and whisk together. Reserve 2 tbsp (30 mL). Marinate salmon in shallow container in remainder of marinade for 45 min, turning every 15 min and frequently re-basting.
2. Broil salmon for about 8 min or until hot in middle (May also bake or grill at 350°F (175°C) for 15 min). Remove once to recoat with marinade.

For Spinach:

1. Place spinach in large nonstick pan with 2 tbsp (30 mL) olive oil and the reserved 2 tbsp (30 mL) of marinade. Cover pan and place on medium high heat. Lift cover to stir every 2–3 min. Turn off heat when spinach begins to wilt and remove cover.

To Complete:

1. Remove salmon from skin (if still present) and serve on wilted spinach.

Notes

This delicious dish pairs well with many of the recipes in this chapter served as side items including brown and wild rice salad, bean salad, fennel salad, Mediterranean quinoa salad, quinoa salad with mint and lime, herb roasted vegetables, roasted balsamic beets, and roasted Italian squash.

Paella

Serves 6–8

Ingredients

2 Pounds (900 g) boneless, skinless chicken breasts, cut into 1-in (2.5 cm) pieces (omit for vegetarian)
1 Pound (450 g) peeled and deveined shrimp (omit for vegetarian)
1 Pound (450 g) scallops (omit for vegetarian)
1 Pound (450 g) vegetarian sausage, Italian or chorizo flavored
2 Cups (500 mL) brown rice
½ Cup (125 mL) extra virgin olive oil
1 Large yellow onion, chopped
4 Cloves garlic, minced
1 Red bell pepper, diced

1 Yellow bell pepper, diced
1 Cup (250 mL) frozen peas, thawed
1 Can (about 15 oz or 425 g) marinated artichoke hearts, halves and quarters
1 Can (about 15 oz or 425 g) diced tomatoes
5 Cups (1,250 mL) vegetable broth
½ Cup (125 mL) chopped fresh parsley leaves
1 tbsp (15 mL) paprika
2 tbsp (10 mL) dried oregano
2 tbsp (10 mL) sea or kosher salt
2 tbsp (10 mL) ground black pepper
1 tbsp (5 mL) red pepper flakes
1 Large pinch saffron threads

Directions

4. Preheat oven to 350°F (175°C).
5. In large skillet over medium high heat, add ¼ cup (60 mL) olive oil and sauté onions and garlic for about 2 min. Add chicken along with paprika, oregano, salt, and black pepper. Continue to cook until chicken starts to brown, then reduce to medium heat.
6. Now add shrimp, scallops, sausage, remainder of olive oil, bell peppers, red pepper flakes, and tomatoes. Gently mix ingredients together and turn off heat.
7. Put rice, vegetable broth, artichokes, peas, and parsley in large Dutch oven or baking dish. Add saffron and gently mix all together. Next, pour entire contents of skillet into rice dish and gently mix until evenly arranged.
8. Cover dish with aluminum foil and bake for 30 min. Remove dish and add additional vegetable broth if dry. Re-cover dish and bake additional 15 min or until rice is soft.

Notes

Paella is one of my favorite dishes, which I learned to cook while living in the Mediterranean. One can make variations on this delicious paella recipe such as choosing just one type of seafood in larger quantities or eliminating all meat and increasing and adding additional seasonal and/or marinated vegetables. Paella is a fun dish to experiment with as the results are almost always flavorful.

Pasta Fagioli

Serves 4

Ingredients

1 Pound (450 g) vegetarian sausage, Italian spiced (Tofurkey is one common brand)

2 tbsp (30 mL) extra virgin olive oil

2 Cans (15 oz or 425 g each) cannellini beans

1 Can (15 oz or 425 g) chopped, stewed tomatoes

1 Small zucchini, chopped

1 Carrot, chopped

1 Onion, chopped

2 Ribs celery, chopped

4 Cloves garlic, minced

2 Quarts (1.9 liters) vegetable stock

8 oz (240 mL) whole wheat penne or shells or rotini pasta

2 Bay leaves

½ tbsp (2.5 mL) rosemary

½ tbsp (2.5 mL) thyme

1 Tbsp (5 mL) oregano

½ tbsp (2.5 mL) red pepper flakes

¼ tbsp (1.25 mL) sea or kosher salt

¼ tbsp (1.25 mL) black pepper

Directions

1. In a large stock pot over medium high heat, add all ingredients except for pasta. Stir occasionally until water starts to boil rapidly, then add pasta and reduce heat to medium.
2. Continue to cook pasta, stirring occasionally, for about 15 min. Turn off heat, remove bay leaves, and serve.

Notes

This is a great recipe to make a double or triple batch of for entertaining or to reheat for several days of healthy leftovers.

Pistachio Dill Salmon

Ingredients

2 lb (490 g) salmon filets

2 tbsp (30 mL) fresh lemon juice

½ Cup (120 mL) dill, chopped
1 Medium sized onion, chopped
1 Cup (250 mL) pistachios (shelled), toasted, and finely chopped
½ Cup (125 mL) extra virgin olive oil
4 tbsp (60 mL) capers
3 Cloves garlic, minced
¼ tbsp sea salt
Pinch of salt and ground black pepper for salmon

Directions

1. Evenly spoon lemon juice onto filets, and then sprinkle with pinch of salt and pepper. Next, broil filets for 8–10 min or until center is hot and flaky.
2. Mix remainder of ingredients in medium sized pot until evenly blended. Place pot over medium low heat and stir constantly for 5 min.
3. When salmon is done, place on serving plates and spoon even amounts of pistachio sauce over each piece.

Notes

This recipe adds a nice tangy, nutty flavor to salmon that enhances the delicious taste of the cooked fish. It pairs well with many of the recipes in this chapter served as side items including arugula salad, brown and wild rice salad, bean salad, fennel salad, Mediterranean quinoa salad, quinoa salad with mint and lime, herb roasted vegetables, roasted beets, and roasted squash.

Pita Pizzas: Red or Green

Serves 4

Ingredients

Both:

6 Large whole wheat pita rounds
2 tbsp (30 mL) extra virgin olive oil

For Red:

1 Can (about 6.5 oz or 190 mL) tomato sauce
1 Red bell pepper, chopped
½ Cup (120 mL) crimini mushrooms, halved
1 Onion, diced

8–10 Kalmata olives, quartered (may substitute marinated artichoke quarters)
½ tbsp dried basil
½ tbsp dried oregano
½ Cup (125 mL) mozzarella cheese
¼ Cup (60 mL) grated Parmesan cheese
Optional: 6 marinated artichoke hearts, quartered

For Green:

⅔ cup (160 mL) pesto sauce
1 Cup (250 mL) cherry or grape tomatoes, halved
10–12 Kalmata olives, halved (may substitute marinated artichoke quarters)
½ Cup (120 mL) crimini mushrooms, halved
1 Can (15 oz or 425 g) white beans, well drained
6 oz (170 g) goat cheese, crumbled

Directions

1. Preheat oven to 425°F (220°C).
2. Place pita rounds on baking sheets and top evenly with olive oil, then top with sauce (pesto or red).
3. Add respective toppings and bake 10 min.

Notes

These flavorful quick pizzas can serve as appetizers or meals. The toppings can be modified based on personal tastes and ingredients on hand.

Quesadillas with Goat Cheese and Black Bean

Serves 4

Ingredients

4 Whole wheat tortillas
2 tbsp (10 mL) extra virgin olive oil
1 Can (15 oz or 425 g) black beans, well drained
1 Red bell pepper, chopped
1 Medium onion, chopped
1 Ripe avocado, sliced lengthwise
½ Cup (250 mL) cilantro, chopped
½ Cup (125 mL) goat cheese

Directions

1. Assemble quesadilla by dividing ingredients evenly on 2 tortillas, then top each with remaining tortillas.
2. In large non-stick skillet add oil and turn on medium heat. Cook one quesadilla at a time for about 3–4 min each side until slightly brown.
3. Cut into wedges and serve.

Notes

Quesadillas are a quick to prepare and nutritious choice for appetizers or whole meals. Scrambled or fried egg whites/egg substitute may be added to make these breakfast quesadillas.

Salmon Burgers

Serves 4

Ingredients

1 Pound salmon filets, skinned and minced with sharp knife (note: may substitute tuna or other firm fish)
1 Green onion, chopped
½ Cup dried whole wheat bread crumbs
2 Egg whites
1 tbsp (15 mL) extra virgin olive oil
1 tbsp (15 mL) Worcestershire sauce
2 tbsp (30 mL) chopped cilantro
2 Cloves garlic, minced
1 tbsp (5 mL) cumin
½ tbsp (2.5 mL) salt and ½ tbsp (2.5 mL) black pepper

Directions

1. Place minced salmon in large bowl, add other ingredients while mixing together with large fork until evenly blended.
2. Shape into 4 patties and cook in non-stick pan with 1 tbsp (15 mL) olive oil added over medium heat for approximately 5 min on each side.
3. Serve on whole grain buns.

Notes

These burgers have a great mix of flavors and are easy to make. They may also be cooked on the grill. Sliced avocado, tomato, lettuce, and seasoned mayonnaise nicely complement these burgers.

Sautéed Fish Provencal

Serves 4

Ingredients

1 Pound of fillets of cod, halibut, sole, or hake, skinned
3 tbsp (45 mL) extra virgin olive oil
1 tbsp (15 mL) capers
8–10 Kalamata olives, quartered
2 Green onions, chopped
½ tbsp (2.5 mL) thyme
1 tbsp (5 mL) basil
8–10 plum or cherry tomatoes quartered
½ tbsp (2.5 mL) sea or kosher salt
½ tbsp (2.5 mL) black pepper

Directions

1. In heavy, non-stick skillet place 2 tbsp (30 mL) olive oil and then place fish fillets. Turn burner to medium heat.
2. After cooking about 2 min, add remainder of olive oil to top of fish and then add remainder of ingredients. Cover skillet and allow to cook for approximately 10 min (about 8 min if fillets are thin), covered continuously. Remove cover and check fish, cook until fish is flaky and then serve immediately.

Notes

This traditional MedDiet fish dish is simple to make and delicious to eat. It is complemented by many of the recipes in this chapter served as side items including arugula salad, brown and wild rice salad, bean salad, fennel salad, Mediterranean quinoa salad, quinoa salad with mint and lime, herb roasted vegetables, roasted beets, and roasted squash.

Smoked Salmon Quesadilla

Serves 4

Ingredients

4 Whole wheat tortillas
4 oz (110 g) smoked salmon
2 tbsp (10 mL) extra virgin olive oil
2 tbsp (30 mL) capers
1 Ripe avocado, peeled, seeded, and sliced lengthwise
1 Red onion, sliced
12 Cherry or plum tomatoes, halved
½ Cup (125 mL) goat cheese

Directions

1. Assemble quesadilla by dividing ingredients evenly on 2 tortillas and then topping each with remaining tortillas.
2. In a large non-stick skillet add oil and turn on medium heat. Cook one quesadilla at a time for about 3–4 min each side until slightly brown.
3. Cut into wedges and serve.

Notes

These flavorful quesadillas combine several classic MedDiet ingredients in a quick to prepare and nutritious choice for appetizers or whole meals. Scrambled or fried egg whites/egg substitute may be added to make these breakfast quesadillas.

Spaghetti with Vegetables and Chicken or Tofu

Serves 4–6

Ingredients

12 oz (350 g) whole wheat spaghetti
1 Jar or can (total about 16 oz or 450 g) marinara (or flavor of choice) pasta sauce

10 Cherry or plum tomatoes, halved
4 tbsp (60 mL) extra virgin olive oil
1 Medium onion, chopped
2 Cloves garlic, minced
1 Yellow bell pepper, chopped
2 Cups cauliflower florets
½ Cup (125 mL) mushrooms, sliced (crimini mushrooms preferred if available)
1 Pound (450 g) boneless skinless chicken breast, cubed; or 1 block firm tofu, cubed
8 oz (225 g) spinach leaves
¼ Cup (60 mL) shredded Parmesan cheese
¼ tbsp (1.25 mL) sea or kosher salt
¼ tbsp (1.25 mL) black pepper
¼ tbsp (1.25 mL) celery salt

Directions

For Spaghetti

1. Cook whole wheat spaghetti per directions on package and drain well.

For Sauce

2. In a large skillet add 2 tbsp (30 mL) olive oil, onion, and garlic and set over medium high heat and sauté until they start to brown, then reduce heat to medium and add yellow pepper, tomatoes, cauliflower, and mushrooms. Stir while cooking for about 5 min. Add spinach, continue to cook until spinach wilts, then add pasta sauce and reduce heat to low, stirring occasionally.
3. In another skillet add 2 tbsp (30 mL) olive oil and chicken or tofu (see section "Tofu: How to Cook") plus salt, pepper, and celery salt. Set over medium high heat and stir occasionally until chicken or tofu browns and then turn off heat.
4. Place pasta in bowls or plates and use ladle or large serving spoon to cover with marinara vegetable sauce and tofu or chicken. Sprinkle with Parmesan cheese.

Notes

This dish contains whole grains, vegetables, fiber, and healthy oils in a pleasing combination. One may choose to add additional pasta sauce or vegetables (I occasionally will add broccoli, carrots, and/or squash depending on my mood) as desired. Pasta dishes such as this make great leftovers for several days so I often double the batch.

Tofu: How to Cook

Ingredients

Tofu

Directions and Notes

Other than simply adding cut tofu to a dish being cooked, there are two basic ways I prepare tofu for use as a meat substitute. Both are described below.

Prepared Standard:

1. Open tofu package, pour out excess water to discard, and remove block of tofu.
2. Place tofu block between two thick, highly absorbent towels. Place a cutting board or similar object on top towel and press with about 10 pounds of weight for approximately 1 min to squeeze out excess water.
3. Place the now squeezed block of tofu onto a cutting board and cut into shapes as called for in recipe, usually triangles or cubes. Thinner shapes will cook firmer.
4. Place cut tofu pieces in large, non-stick skillet with spices, about 2 tbsp of oil (olive, canola, or peanut), and 2 tbsp of marinade per block.
5. Sauté tofu over medium high heat until each side is golden brown.
6. Prepared tofu may now be used as desired in dish.

Prepared Dry Style (Generally Firmer):

1. Follow steps 1 and 2 as above.
2. Freeze block of tofu airtight container for at least 4 h and up to two weeks.
3. When ready to cook, remove frozen tofu from container and microwave in shallow, microwave safe dish at medium power for about 5 min, checking occasionally, until block is soft enough to cut. Pour off excess water and repeat step 2 above.
4. Place block of tofu onto cutting board and cut into shapes as called for in recipe. Thinner shapes will cook firmer.
5. Place cut tofu pieces in large, non-stick skillet with spices, about 2 tbsp of flavorful oil, and 2 tbsp of marinade per block.
6. Sauté tofu over medium high heat until each side is golden brown.
7. Prepared tofu may now be used as desired in dish.

Soups and Stews

Carrot and Ginger Soup

Serves 6

Ingredients

2 tbsp (30 mL) extra virgin olive oil
1 Cup (250 mL) diced onion
½ Cup (125 mL) diced celery
¼ Cup (60 mL) minced ginger
1 tbsp (15 mL) minced garlic
½ Pound (225 g) carrots, peeled and roughly chopped
5 Cups (1,500 mL) vegetable or chicken stock
1 tbsp (5 mL) salt
½ tbsp (5 mL) freshly ground white pepper
1 Bay leaf
1 Cup (250 mL) plain Greek yogurt
3 tbsp (45 mL) chopped chives, for garnish

Directions

1. Add the olive oil to a large stockpot and heat over medium-high heat. Add the onion and celery and cook for about 4 min, until the onion is translucent. Add the ginger and garlic to the pot and cook for about 30 seconds. Add the carrots, stirring occasionally, and cook until the carrots are slightly caramelized, 7–8 min. Add the stock, salt, pepper, and bay leaf, bring to a boil, and then reduce heat to a simmer. Cook for 20–25 min, until the carrots are soft.
2. Remove the stockpot from the heat and take out the bay leaf. Using an immersion blender, puree the soup. (Or, let the coup cool slightly and puree in a food processor or blender.) Season to taste with salt and pepper.
3. Return the pot to the burner and reheat the soup over medium heat, being careful to keep in from boiling. Ladle into serving bowls and garnish with the remaining yogurt and chopped chives.

Notes

This flavorful soup pairs well with salads, sandwiches, and fish dishes.

Gazpacho

Serves 4–6

Ingredients

2 Green bell peppers, quartered
1 Red bell pepper, quartered
1 Large onion, quartered
3 Cloves garlic, peeled and split
2 Celery stalks, halved
3 Medium tomatoes, skinned and cored
1 Large cucumber, skinned and cut into 4 pieces
24 oz (700 mL) tomato juice
½ tbsp (2.5 mL) Tabasco® sauce (double to make highly spicy)
1 tbsp (5 mL) lemon juice
⅓ Cup (80 mL) extra virgin olive oil
2 tbsp (30 mL) white wine vinegar
1 tbsp (5 mL) ground cumin seed
2 tbsp (30 mL) fresh cilantro leaves
¼ tbsp (1.25 mL) kosher or sea salt
¼ tbsp (1.25 mL) ground black pepper (double to make highly spicy)

Directions

1. In blender add 1 cup of tomato juice. Then, one at a time, add each vegetable and spice, pulsing until blended. Add remainder of tomato juice as needed to maintain liquidity.
2. Refrigerate for at least 2 h. Serve in chilled bowls.

Notes

This traditional Spanish soup is great in the summer (spring, fall, and winter too) and works well with both casual and more formal lunches and dinners. Nice complements to gazpacho include crusty, multi-grain bread, a freshly made sandwich, or a seasonal green salad. Popular gazpacho variations include adding avocado and/or grilled seafood to the bowl.

Lentil and Brown Rice Soup

Serves 4

Ingredients

1 Cup (250 mL) dried lentils
½ Cup (125 mL) brown rice
6 Cups (1.5 liters) vegetable stock
2 Cans (15 oz or 425 g each) chopped tomatoes with juice
¼ Cup (60 mL) extra virgin olive oil
1 Medium onion, chopped
2 Stalks celery, chopped
2 Carrots, chopped
1 Zucchini, chopped
1 Cup (250 mL) cherry or plum tomatoes, halved
4 Cloves garlic, minced
½ tbsp (2.5 mL) thyme
½ tbsp (2.5 mL) oregano
1 tbsp (5 mL) dried basil
1 Bay leaf
½ tbsp (2.5 mL) sea or kosher salt
1 tbsp (5 mL) black pepper

Directions

1. In large pot, add olive oil and turn to medium high heat. Sautee onion and garlic for 5 min, then turn to medium heat and add celery, carrots, zucchini, and cherry or plum tomatoes. Cook 5 min longer while stirring frequently.
2. Add vegetable stock, cans of chopped tomatoes, lentils, brown rice, thyme, oregano, basil, bay leaf, salt, and pepper. Adjust heat to low simmer and keep covered, stirring occasionally and cook for 35–45 min longer.

Notes

This is a great dish to double or triple the recipe for large gatherings or to have leftovers for several days.

Red Chili with Three Beans

Serves 4–6

Ingredients

1 Can (about 15 oz or 425 g) black beans, drained
1 Can (about 15 oz or 425 g) pinto beans, drained
1 Can (about 15 oz or 425 g) red kidney beans, drained
1 Can (about 15 oz or 425 g) corn
3 Cans (about 15 oz or 425 g each) stewed tomatoes
1 Green bell pepper, diced
2 Stalks celery, diced
3 Cloves garlic, minced
1 tbsp (15 mL) extra virgin olive oil
1 Onion diced
2 tbsp (30 mL) chili powder
1 tbsp (15 mL) ground cumin
1 tbsp (5 mL) oregano
2 tbsp (10 mL) paprika
½ tbsp (2.5 mL) black pepper
½ tbsp (2.5 mL) cayenne
Salt to taste
Optional: chopped meat substitute or diced chicken, sautéed in oil until browned before adding.

Directions

1. Sauté onion and garlic in olive oil in large stockpot.
2. Add additional ingredients and spices and stir gently to blend.
3. Simmer on medium or lower heat for at least 30 min, adding additional water and spices to taste.

Notes

This chili recipe may be doubled or tripled for larger gatherings or to have enough for several days of leftovers.

Seafood Stew

Serves 4–6

Ingredients

½ Pound (225 g) shrimp, peeled and deveined
½ Pound (225 g) white fish, such as cod, haddock or halibut, cubed
½ Pound (225 g) scallops
½ Pound (225 g) crab meat or imitation crabmeat
1 Large onion, chopped
1 Green bell pepper, chopped
1 Carrot, diced
2 Stalks celery, chopped
2 Cloves garlic, minced
2 tbsp (30 mL) extra virgin olive oil
½ Cup (125 mL) frozen corn kernels
½ Cup (125 mL) fresh parsley, finely chopped
2 Cans (about 15 oz or 425 g each) vegetable broth
1 Can (about 15 oz or 425 g) stewed tomato
1 tbsp (5 mL) oregano
1 tbsp (5 mL) thyme
½ tbsp (2.5 mL) crushed red pepper flakes
¼ tbsp (1.25 mL) allspice
2 Cups (500 mL) uncooked brown rice
1 Cup (250 mL) water
½ tbsp (2.5 mL) sea or kosher salt
½ tbsp (2.5 mL) black pepper
1 Bay leaf

Directions

1. In large stock pot, add oil, onion, and garlic. Sautee over medium-high heat for 3–5 min, reduce to medium heat and add green pepper, carrot, and celery. Cook for about 2–3 min more, stirring frequently. Then add remainder of ingredients. Simmer covered, stirring occasionally and adjusting temperature as needed for about 45 min or until rice is tender. Additional water or vegetable broth may be added for a soupier consistency.
2. Serve in bowls.

Notes

This stew recipe is great for doubling or even tripling the batch for large gatherings or for providing several days of leftovers. It goes great with a side of rustic, multi-grain bread.

Three Bean Italian Soup

Serves 4

Ingredients

1 Can (15 oz or 425 mL) white beans
1 Can (15 oz or 425 mL) red kidney beans
1 Can (15 oz or 425 mL) pinto beans or black beans
1 Can (15 oz or 425 mL) stewed tomatoes
2 Cans (30 oz or 850 mL) vegetable broth
2 tbsp (30 mL) extra virgin olive oil
1 tbsp (5 mL) basil
1 tbsp (5 mL) oregano
2 Tbsp (30 mL) balsamic vinegar
½ tbsp (2.5 mL) black pepper
2 Bay leaves
Sea or kosher salt to taste

Directions

1. Combine all ingredients in a large pot and bring to a slow boil over medium heat at medium heat, stirring occasionally. Reduce heat to medium low, cover, and simmer for 10–15 min.
2. Remove bay leaves and serve.

Notes

This is a quick, simple, and flavorful recipe that reheats well for leftovers. The ingredients may be doubled or tripled as desired.

White Chili with Chicken

Serves 6

Ingredients

3 cans (about 15 oz or 425 g each) white kidney or cannellini beans, drained
4 cans (about 15 oz or 425 g each) vegetable broth
1 Pound (450 g) boneless, skinless chicken breast, cut into 1-inch (2 cm) pieces
(For vegetarian may omit or substitute tofu, see "Tofu, How to Cook")
3 Onions, chopped
1 Red bell pepper, chopped
1 Cup mushrooms, sliced (use crimini mushrooms for optimal flavor)
1 tbsp extra virgin olive oil
3 Cloves garlic, minced
1 piece ginger root, about 2 in (5 cm), peeled and minced
1 Jalapeno pepper, stemmed, seeded, and finely chopped
1 Bay leaf
1 tbsp (5 mL) dried oregano
2 Tbsp (10 mL) cumin
3 tbsp (45 mL) extra virgin olive oil
½ tbsp (2.5 mL) black or white pepper
1 Cup fresh cilantro leaves
Salt to taste

Directions

1. In large stock pot, sauté onions and garlic in 2 tbsp (30 mL) olive oil over medium high heat until just start to brown. Reduce to medium heat and add mushrooms, ginger, jalapeno, and red bell pepper. Continue to cook, stirring occasionally, until vegetables begin to soften.
2. Add broth, beans, and spices and stir until blended. Then add bay leaf.
3. In a separate frying pan, add olive oil and chicken and sauté over medium high heat for about 3 or 4 min until outside starts to brown, then turn off heat and add chicken and any of the remain oil and juices to the pot.
4. Now bring entire mixture to boil, then cover and reduce heat to a low simmer for 30 min or longer, stirring occasionally. Remove bay leaf and serve.

Notes

I love this healthy and unique chili recipe. The recipe may be doubled or tripled for large gatherings or to have enough for several days of leftovers. It reheats very well.

Salads and Sides

Arugula Salad

Serves 4

Ingredients

4 Cups (1,000 mL) baby arugula leaves
1 Medium red onion, sliced
1 Cup (250 mL) cherry tomatoes, halved
1 Avocado, peeled, seeded and sliced
½ Cup (125 mL) walnut halves and quarters
4 oz (110 g) crumbled goat cheese or grated Parmesan cheese
3 tbsp (45 mL) balsamic vinegar
2 tbsp (30 mL) extra virgin olive oil
Pinch of sea salt and ground black pepper

Directions

1. Combine all ingredients except avocado in a large bowl and toss together.
2. Serve salad on plates and top with sliced avocado.

Notes

This easy-to-make salad can be used as a side for nearly any lunch or dinner entrée. It also may be made more substantial by topping with cottage cheese, broiled fish, or tuna or chicken salad.

Bean Salad

Serves 4

Ingredients

2 Cups (500 mL) cooked dried beans (black, white, or lima beans work well)
2 Cups (500 mL) Roma or cherry tomatoes, halved
2 Stalks celery, halved lengthwise then coarsely chopped
1 Cucumber, chopped
¼ Cup (60 mL) green onions, chopped
2 Cloves garlic, minced
10 Kalmata olives, pitted and halved
½ Cup fresh parsley, chopped
¼ Cup (60 mL) extra virgin olive oil
1 tbsp (15 mL) lemon juice
4 oz or ½ cup (125 g) feta cheese, crumbled
½ tbsp (2.5 mL) ground cumin
½ tbsp (2.5 mL) sea or kosher salt
½ tbsp (2.5 mL) fresh ground black pepper

Directions

1. Cook dried beans per package instructions and drain well.
2. In a large salad bowl combine beans and remainder of ingredients and toss until evenly mixed. May be refrigerated prior to serving if a chilled salad is desired.

Notes

This recipe serves as a flavorful side accompaniment to nearly any Mediterranean dish. It also works well for picnics and potlucks.

Brown and Wild Rice, California Walnuts, and Dried Cranberry Salad

Serves 4 entrée sized and 6–8 as side item

Ingredients

2 Cups (500 mL) coarsely chopped California walnuts
4 Cups (1,000 mL) water
1 tbsp (5 mL) salt
2 Cups (500 mL) brown rice and wild rice blend
2 Garlic cloves, minced
2 tbsp (10 mL) minced orange zest
4 tbsp (20 mL) grainy Dijon mustard
4 tbsp (60 mL) orange juice concentrate
½ Cup (125 mL) sherry vinegar (may substitute white wine vinegar)
1 Cup (250 mL) olive oil
1 Cup (250 mL) dried cranberries
1 Red pepper, quartered lengthwise, thinly sliced
6 Green onions, thinly sliced
1 Cup (250 mL) snow peas, sliced ¼ in (0.5 cm) on the diagonal

Directions

1. In dry skillet, toast walnuts over medium-high heat for 1–2 min or until lightly browned. In medium saucepan, bring water and salt to boil. Add rice, stir well, cover and reduce heat to simmer.
2. Cook for 40–45 min or until rice is tender and all water has been absorbed. Remove from heat. Let stand for 10 min. In small bowl, combine garlic, orange zest, and mustard; blend well. Whisk in orange juice concentrate and vinegar. Slowly whisk in oil and salt. Transfer cooked rice to large bowl. Add half the orange mixture and toss gently to coat well. Cool to room temperature.
3. Add walnuts, cranberries, red pepper, green onions, and snow peas just before serving. Toss. Add remaining dressing to lightly coat vegetables. Toss again and serve.

   Recipe courtesy California Walnuts, www.walnuts.org.

Notes

This flavorful dish is a personal favorite and may be served as either an entrée or as a side item, pairing very well with almost all foods. It is also excellent for potlucks, picnics, and tailgating.

Curried Tuna Salad

Serves 4

Ingredients

2 Cans (about 12 oz, or 340 g) tuna, drained
2 tbsp (30 mL) canola or olive oil mayonnaise
2 tbsp (20 mL) fat-free yogurt
2 Stalks celery, finely chopped
1 Red bell pepper, finely chopped
1 Small onion, finely chopped
2 Cups (500 mL) seedless grapes, quartered
½ Cup (125 mL) walnuts, cashews, or pecans, coarsely chopped
1 tbsp (5 mL) yellow mustard
2 tbsp (10 mL) curry powder
1 tbsp garam masala
¼ tbsp kosher or sea salt

Directions

1. In large mixing bowl, combine drained tuna and remainder of ingredients except for grapes. Mix to evenly combine; then add grapes and gently mix until evenly distributed.
2. Serve immediately or refrigerate covered for 30 min to 1 h and serve chilled.

Notes

This versatile tuna salad may also be used for traditional sandwiches, pita pockets, wraps, pasta salads, or topping green salads. One may substitute salmon or chicken for tuna as a variation.

Fennel, White Bean and Walnut Salad

Serves 4

Ingredients

1 Fennel bulb
1 Can, about 15 oz. (425 g) white beans (cannellini or white navy), drained and rinsed
½ Cup (125 mL) shredded carrots
¼ Cup (60 mL) dried currants
¾ Cup (185 mL) toasted California walnut pieces

Dressing:

½ Cup (125 mL) extra virgin olive oil
¼ Cup (60 mL) white wine vinegar
1 tbsp (15 mL) Dijon mustard
¼ Cup (60 mL) mixed, chopped herbs (parsley, chives, tarragon)
Salt and pepper to taste

Directions

1. Thinly slice fennel and place in large bowl with beans, carrots and currants.
2. In a small bowl, whisk together dressing ingredients and pour over bean and fennel mixture.
3. Toss to combine. Sprinkle walnuts on top and serve.

Notes

This recipe makes a salad that may be served as a light entrée or as a flavorful side to nearly any MedDiet dish.
    Recipe courtesy California Walnuts, www.walnuts.org.

Green Bean Salad with Walnuts

Ingredients

1 Cup (250 mL) green beans, trimmed
4 tbsp (60 mL) chopped walnuts
4 tbsp (20 mL) walnut oil (or olive oil)
2 tbsp (10 mL) red wine vinegar
2 tbsp (10 mL) Dijon mustard

4 tbsp (60 mL) finely chopped fresh parsley
½ Cup (125 mL) fresh dill, chopped
4 tbsp (60 mL) chopped red onion
Salt and pepper to taste

Directions

1. Bring a large pot of water with a steamer basket to a boil, add green beans and steam for 5 min. Transfer to a serving bowl.
2. Toast the walnuts in a small dry skillet over medium heat until they become fragrant, about 2 min, and then transfer to a small bowl. Add the parsley and onion to the walnuts and stir to continue.
3. In another small bowl, whisk together the oil, vinegar, and mustard.
4. Toss the dressing with the green beans, top with the walnut mixture, and season with salt and pepper.
5. Serve warm or at room temperature.

Notes

This recipe does makes a delicious side item that goes well with more formal meals served warm and more casual meals served cool. The cooled green bean salad is great for picnics.

Recipe courtesy California Walnuts, www.walnuts.org.

Herb Roasted Vegetables

Serves 4–6

Ingredients

Choose mix of 3, 4, or more vegetables from:
2 Cups (500 mL) broccoli florets
2 Cups (500 mL) cauliflower florets
1 Large onion, cut into large chunks
1 Pound (450 g) new potatoes, quartered
1 Pound (450 g) baby carrots
1 Pound (450 g) asparagus
1 Large red bell pepper, seeded and cut into large strips

Other Ingredients:

1 Cup (250 mL) extra virgin olive oil

1 tbsp (30 mL) dried rosemary
1 tbsp (15 mL) herbes de Provence
1 tbsp (5 mL) kosher or sea salt

Directions

1. Preheat oven to 350°F (175°C).
2. In large baking dish, place mix of 3 or 4 vegetables (or larger volume of single vegetable) and coat with olive oil, rosemary, herbes de Provence, and salt. Mix together with metal spatula or serving spoon to evenly coat.
3. Bake for about 40 min, removing every 10 min to stir. If vegetables start to brown, reduce heat to avoid burning.

Notes

Seasonal vegetables are one of the highlights of a MedDiet. This is a quick way to prepare vegetables for serving them as a side item, as a topping for green salads, or as a meal themselves. One may also mix the olive oil, rosemary, herbes de Provence, and salt together and coat vegetables prior to grilling.

Mediterranean Chicken Salad

Serves 4

Ingredients

½ Pound (225 g) boneless, skinless chicken breast, cooked and chopped (for vegetarians, may substitute 1 can welldrained white beans for chicken)
1 Small onion, chopped
2 Celery stalks, chopped
1 Cup (250 mL) grated carrots
2 Cups (500 mL) cherry or grape tomatoes, halved
2 tbsp (30 mL) capers
1 Cup (250 mL) kalamata olives, halved
¼ Cup (60 mL) feta cheese, crumbled
1 tbsp (15 mL) lemon juice
1 tbsp (15 mL) Dijon mustard
2 tbsp (30 mL) extra virgin olive oil
1 Cup (250 mL) plain Greek yogurt
½ Cup (125 mL) chopped walnuts

¼ tbsp (1.25 mL) kosher or sea salt
¼ tbsp (1.25 mL) ground black pepper

Directions

1. In large mixing bowl, combine all ingredients except for tomatoes and mix until evenly combined, then add tomatoes and gently mix until evenly distributed.
2. Serve immediately or refrigerate covered and serve chilled.

Notes

This versatile salad may be used for traditional sandwiches, pita pockets, wraps, pasta salads, or topping green salads. One may substitute salmon or tuna for a variation.

Mediterranean Quinoa Salad

Serves 8

Ingredients

2 Cups (500 mL) dry quinoa
4 Cups (1000 mL) hot water
2 Cups (500 mL) peas, lightly cooked fresh or frozen
1 Medium red onion, diced
1 Red bell pepper, seeded, cored, and diced
1 Green bell pepper, seeded, cored, and diced
½ Cup (125 mL) black olives, sliced and pitted
¼ Cup (62.5 mL) fresh parsley, chopped
¼ Cup (62.5 mL) fresh dill, chopped
1 Cup (500 mL) raisins
¼ Cup (62.5 mL) pine nuts, toasted
½ Cup (125 mL) vinaigrette dressing

Directions

1. In a large saucepan, bring 4 cups hot water and 2 cups quinoa to a boil. Cover and cook over low heat for 15 min or until all the water is absorbed. Fluff with a fork and cool.

2. When quinoa and peas are cool, place in a large bowl and add all remaining ingredients except pine nuts. Toss with a cup of vinaigrette dressing or try the dressing that follows. Taste and adjust for seasonings. Add more dressing if desired.
3. Garnish with pine nuts toasted until golden in a dry skillet.
4. Serve warm or cover and chill up to 4 h.

White Vinagrette Dressing

¼ Cup (62.5 mL) white balsamic vinegar
1 tbsp (5 mL) sugar
1 tbsp (5 mL) Dijon mustard
2 Cloves garlic, finely chopped
½ Cup (125 mL) olive oil
¼ Cup plus 2 tbsp (72.5 mL) dry white wine
Freshly ground pepper
Salt

Directions

Whisk together vinegar, sugar, mustard and chopped garlic in a bowl. Slowly drizzle in the olive oil and wine, whisking until well blended. Adjust seasonings to taste.

Notes

This is a versatile salad that is excellent on its own or as a side dish. It also works well for potlucks and picnics.
    Recipe courtesy Bob's Red Mill Natural Foods www.bobsredmill.com.

Quinoa Salad with Mint and Lime

Serves 8

Ingredients

2 Cups (500 mL) dry quinoa
4 Cups (1,000 mL) water
2 Cups (500 mL) fresh or frozen (thawed) corn
1 Cup (250 mL) chopped scallions
1 Cup (250 mL) chopped fresh mint

1 Cup (250 mL) slivered almonds
1 Cup (250 mL) fresh diced mango; may substitute ½ cup (125 mL) dried apricots
¼ Cup (60 mL) extra virgin olive oil
2 tbsp (30 mL) agave nectar or honey
4 tbsp (60 mL) fresh lime juice
1–2 tbsp (5–10 mL) tamari added to taste
3 tbsp (15 mL) sea or kosher salt
½ tbsp (2.5 mL) white pepper

Directions

1. Rinse and drain quinoa.
2. In a medium saucepan, bring quinoa and water to boil and cover, simmering for about 12 min or until all the water is absorbed. Transfer quinoa to a large bowl, fluff, and allow to cool.
3. In a small bowl, mix olive oil, honey or agave, lime juice, salt, pepper, and tamari.
4. Add corn, mint, scallions, almonds, and apricots or mango to quinoa and mix in dressing. Serve room temperature or cover and chill up to 4 h.

Notes

I love this versatile side dish that can also be used for extra flavor instead of rice or pasta for the base of fish dishes, curries, stir fries, and poultry. It also works well for potlucks and picnics and makes easy leftovers for several days.

Roasted Balsamic Beets

Serves 4

Ingredients

3 ½ Pounds assorted small beets, peeled and cut in half
½ Cup (120 mL) olive oil
1 tbsp balsamic vinegar
1 tbsp fresh or dried rosemary
1 tbsp (5 mL) sea or kosher salt

Directions

1. Preheat oven to 400°F.
2. In a large mixing bowl, coat beets in olive oil, and rosemary.
3. Place beets in casserole dish, cover, and bake at 400° for 35–40 min.
4. Uncover, toss beets in dish, and drizzle with salt and balsamic vinegar. Bake for 5 additional minutes. Serve hot.

Notes

This beet dish melds the earthy flavor of beets (and any other vegetable you choose to prepare with this flavorful marinade) with the tangy flavor of balsamic vinegar. It creates a perfect side for nearly any dish and is one of my favorite ways to prepare vegetables.

Rustic Tuna on Greens

Serves 4

Ingredients

2 Cans (about 12 oz, or 340 g) tuna, drained
1 Pound (450 g) asparagus
1 Red onion, sliced
8–10 Kalamata olives, quartered
2 Cups (500 mL) cherry or plum tomatoes, halved
2 tbsp (30 mL) capers
½ tbsp (2.5 mL) dried basil
1 Can (15 oz or 425 g) garbanzo beans, well drained
1 Cup (250 mL) artichoke hearts halves and quarters, marinated
1 tbsp (15 mL) extra virgin olive oil
¼ tbsp sea or kosher salt
¼ tbsp ground black pepper
¼ Cup (mL) balsamic vinaigrette

Or, Make Own Vinaigrette with:

3 tbsp (45 mL) balsamic vinegar
3 tbsp (45 mL) extra virgin olive oil
2 Cloves garlic, minced

1 tbsp (5 mL) Dijon mustard
1 tbsp (5 mL) lemon juice
1 tbsp (5 mL) oregano

Directions

1. In medium nonstick skillet, sauté onion and asparagus in 1 tbsp (15 mL) olive oil over medium heat for about 5 min. Add tomatoes, capers, beans, olives, artichokes, salt and pepper, and heat approximately 3 min longer. Turn off heat.
2. In separate small bowl, combine balsamic vinegar, oregano, olive oil, garlic, Dijon, and lemon juice.
3. On bed of mixed greens, add tuna with a fork to evenly distribute, add asparagus mixture, then drizzle dressing over salad.

Notes

This is a great combination of MedDiet flavors that I make frequently. I love it served with warmed rustic bread dipped in extra virgin olive oil. As a variation, one may substitute fresh tuna, salmon, or chicken for the canned tuna.

Desserts

Chilled Fruit and Yogurt Bowl

Serves 8

Ingredients

6 Cups (1,500 mL) of assorted fruits of choice—including banana, blackberries, blueberries, cantaloupe, kiwi, mango, raspberries, seedless grapes, strawberries—sliced or cubed
2 Cups (500 mL) fat-free plain yogurt
2 tbsp (30 mL) orange juice
2 tbsp (30 mL) lemon juice
1 tbsp (5 mL) poppy seeds
¼ tbsp (1.25 mL) ginger
½ tbsp nutmeg
Optional: ¼ cup (60 mL) shredded coconut

Directions

1. In medium bowl, mix orange juice, lemon juice, poppy seeds, ginger, and nutmeg. Then add yogurt and stir until blended.
2. In large bowl, place fruit and then gradually add yogurt mix while stirring gently to evenly coat fruit.
3. Refrigerate for 1 h and serve chilled.

Notes

This dish is great as a healthy dessert alternative and can be served in casual or more formal dishes depending on the situation. It is also great for picnics, potlucks, and keeping in the refrigerator as a quick snack. Doubling or tripling the recipe in an extra large bowl allows for nutritious sides, desserts, and snacks for several days.

Fruit, Granola, and Yogurt Parfaits

Serves 4

Ingredients

½ Cup (125 mL) low fat vanilla yogurt
¼ Cup (60 mL) fat-free cream cheese
1 tbsp (15 mL) honey
¼ tbsp (1.25 mL) ground cinnamon
2 Kiwifruit, halved lengthwise and sliced
1 Medium banana, sliced
1 Medium orange, sliced
1 ½ Cup (375 mL) frozen berries, thawed and drained
1 Cup natural granola

Directions

1. In a small mixing bowl, combine the yogurt, cream cheese, honey, and cinnamon. Beat with an electric mixer on medium speed till combined; chill.
2. In a small bowl, stir fruit together. Divide one-third of the fruit mixture among four parfait glasses or wine goblets. Spoon about half of each of the cream cheese mixture and granola atop fruit; repeat layers. Top with remaining third of fruit. Serve immediately.

Notes

This recipe makes a fairly sweet dessert that goes well after a highly spiced or savory meal. I simply eliminate the honey or substitute plain yogurt for the vanilla yogurt to reduce sweetness and have a more breakfast-granola style dish for the mornings.

Recipe courtesy Bob's Red Mill Natural Foods, www.bobsredmill.com.

Simple Fruit Crisp

Serves 6–8

Ingredients

10 oz (285 g) fresh or frozen blueberries
16 oz (450 g) fresh or frozen peaches, sliced
¼ (60 mL) Cup apple juice
½ Cup (125 mL) almonds
½ Cup (125 mL) oats
1 Cup (250 mL) pitted dates
½ tbsp (1.25 mL) cinnamon
2 tbsp (30 mL) apple juice
¼ Cup (60 mL) pecans

Directions

1. Preheat oven to 300°F (150°C). Place blueberries in the bottom of an 8-in. (20 cm) square baking dish. Place peaches on top of blueberries. Drizzle ¼ cup (60 mL) apple juice over fruit.
2. In a food processor, puree almonds, oats, dates, and cinnamon. After 1 min add apple juice and continue to puree. Evenly spread mixture over fruit and top with pecans.
3. Bake uncovered for about 40–45 min. Cut into six pieces. Serve warm or allow to cool.

Notes

This is a healthy dessert alternative loaded with flavor and nutrients. If using frozen fruit, make sure it is completely thawed and drained of excess water before using.

Recipe courtesy of Produce for Better Health Foundation, www.fruitsandveggiesmorematters.org.

ERRATUM TO

Chapter 19
Recipes

E. Zacharias, *The Mediterranean Diet: A Clinician's Guide for Patient Care*,
DOI 10.1007/978-1-4614-3326-2_19, © Springer Science+Business Media, LLC 2012

DOI 10.1007/978-1-4614-3326-2_20

The publisher regrets that in chapter 19 "Recipes", the abbreviation for teaspoon ("tsp") had mistakenly printed as "tbsp" in some of the recipes. Due to this error please note when reading the recipes:

The metric units remain correct. Please use the metric units in recipes with "tbsp" listed to ensure you are using the intended amount of ingredient. The following conversions may be helpful:

1.25ml = 1/4 tsp; 2.5ml = 1/2 tsp; 5ml = 1 tsp; 10ml = 2 tsp;
15ml = 1 tbsp; 30ml = 2 tbsp

The online version of the original chapter can be found at
http://dx.doi.org/10.1007/978-1-4614-3326-2_19

Index

1840496R00141

Made in the USA
San Bernardino, CA
07 February 2013